Divine Healing

For the Individual and for the Church

Bruce Williams

with

Alta Ada Williams

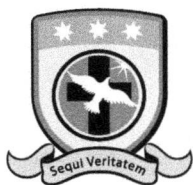

Sequi Veritatem

Lititz Institute

Publishing Division

Published by Lititz Institute Publishing Division
PO Box 3310, Sequim WA 98382
www.lititzinstitute.org

Printed in the United States of America

Authors Edition November 2017

Library of Congress Cataloging-in-Publication Data

Williams, R. Bruce

>Divine Healing for the Individual and for the Church
>Richard Bruce Williams

>p.   cm.

>ISBN 978-0-9820014-6-2   (paprerback)

>1. Study of when God Heals 2. Study of how God Heals
>3. Study of God's Character
>4. Study of the Spiritual decline of the Church
>5. God's solutions for a spiritually ill Church

>1. Title

All Scripture quotations are teken from The Authorized King James Version of the Holy Bible.

This book is dedicated with grateful thanks to my best friend, and my sweet wife, Alta Ada Williams.

This book is also dedicated to Bishop Willie L. Cage of Hammond, Louisiana.

The book would not have been possible without the loving discussions and sharing the three of us have on a regular basis, regarding what God is revealing in His Holy Scriptures and in His whisperings to each of us. Bishop is so kind and gracious to spend his time with us. He has been implementing many of the concepts in this book in his local church; as a result there are now frequent healing miracles.

We have learned much from each other regarding the work of the Holy Spirit in teaching us and revealing our Lord Jesus Christ in all of His great Glory. He is the King of Kings and the Lord of Lords. How excellent is He in all the heavens and in all the earth; His great name is to be praised.

Bishop Cage is the founding Pastor of God's Tabernacle of Deliverance Church of God in Christ in Hammond LA, affectionately called (GTOD), a thriving ministry on the cutting edge. He has served in various capacities with the Church of God in Christ, including the Executive Committee for the National Leadership Convention, Administrative Assistant in the Greater New Orleans Jurisdiction and Superintendent of the Deliverance District. In 2016, Bishop Cage was consecrated as the Jurisdictional Prelate of South Central Louisiana Ecclesiastical Jurisdiction by the Presiding Bishop of the Churches of God in Christ, Inc., Bishop Charles Edward Blake.

No one needs to be thanked more than our Lord God who has lovingly guided the writing of this text. It is not inerrant, Our God is the God and Father of the Lord Jesus Christ.

Table of Contents

Chapter Title

Foundational Concepts for Understanding God and the Bible

Chapter One

Setting the Stage

We are going to talk about the limits and expectations the reader can have for this book.

1. We are going to talk about healing that God (we will define which God) sometimes gives for physical health issues. We are not God and can guarantee no results for any other person approaching God for healing. We are not an intermediary for God, and no one should ever let anyone else take this role. No one should ever be under the control of another person regarding seeking God for healing, or be told by someone else what God is saying.

2. This book is about healing for spiritual illness and physical illness in both individuals and in the Church as the body of the Lord Jesus Christ. The Church, defined as the body of the Lord Jesus Christ, is not parallel to those entities in society which bear the label of a church, although obviously there is considerable overlap.

3. We are going to try to give the reader ways that Scripture indicates to us as being able to increase the likelihood that God will heal him.

4. God operates by His rules regarding when He will give physical healing and these are not in any specific situation ones which any person can interpret or predict. Our comments are general ones for the people of the Church. We will use a capital C when referring to the Church constituted of the body of the Lord Jesus Christ. Generally spiritual healing and physical healing are both needed when a physical illness or infirmity is present.

5. For those who are not in the Church there are no instructions regarding healing in God's written word, the Bible. We note that God frequently healed those people when He walked on the earth during His advent as the Lord Jesus Christ, and that His character is such that he heals, He is compassionate, He is kind, and He is merciful.

6. Many people think they are in the Church; and they are not, having been deceived by evil spirits at the time of an earlier commitment to God. These people have no written guarantees from God.

7. God actually commands those in the Church to be healed by Him; but this is a complex issue, and we try to address it in the book. In each individual situation there are so many variables, which are known only to God and perhaps to the person seeking healing, that no one, including the seeker of healing, can guarantee any specific result. Our comments in the book are general ones. We do try to address how people can work with God to be healed, but there is a lot of deception by evil spirits and by the flesh (pride) so that it can be quite difficult to know what God will grant.

8. A key for knowing what God will do is to be able to communicate with Him, so we focus much of the book on how to develop reliable communications with God. This does not come easily, and it does not come without time and effort. One learns to communicate well with God only as he gains a deep knowledge of the Bible taught by the Holy Spirit and not by man alone. This knowledge will be readily discernable by others in authority in the Church.

9. No one should accept the word of any prophetic statement regarding being healed. One can be encouraged by this but he still has to deal directly with God. Absolutely no other person can ever, ever, speak authoritatively for God in each and every situation. Some prophets are more ma-

ture and reliable than others, but knowing how to choose the better ones takes spiritual maturity.

This whole issue of getting divine healing would be easy to address were it not for two enemies which oppose a person being healed by God: the flesh (defined later) and evil spirits. These two agents, acting separately and jointly, can cause a lot of confusion. As a physician Bruce has seen many people who thought they had been healed by God, stopped treatments, were too proud to get tested, and experienced disastrous results. No one wants to see this kind of situation. Pride is one of the major spiritual illnesses, and without getting this healed one will have a very difficult time communicating with God. He will not know how to understand the origin of his thoughts.

10. As a rule one should seek God's healing only as he continues to work with his physician and with experienced counsel who is spiritually mature and in leadership in his local church. One should never stop vital medication or other treatment without agreement from his physician and his spiritual leaders. People think that walking in faith is important with God; and so it is. Faith is not blind trust or proudly making a stance in the view of others. Faith is knowing absolutely when God speaks to him and can come only as one learns to communicate with God. It is not easy for a proud person to develop this true faith. If a person has the slightest doubt about what God has said in any situation, then he does not have true faith and should not expect God to fulfill any commitment. In this case a person should absolutely continue under medical care for his health problems. God actually regards it as sin to do otherwise (Romans 14:23).

11. When God heals, there is no doubt in the individual receiving it and in others observing him. A physician will be able to say that healing has taken place or that it has started. The physician may not wish to credit God but that

is not why one goes to a physician; one wants and respects the technical and professional medical advice he gets. The healing will be obvious to the physician. No one should ever be too proud to have a healing authenticated, even if not correctly attributed to the right source.

We hope that setting this stage will be of help for keeping a proper perspective as one proceeds through this book.

The Purpose for this Book

We are writing this book to speak to people who are burdened in any way by their physical and emotional situations. There are so many people who are hurting inside in our Western societies. Some become defeated; others become hardened; but few are able to change their circumstances for the better. There are two major parts to a man—his spirit (inner man) and his physical body (flesh). The two considered overall are termed in the Bible a soul. The spirit is an inner man that is shaped like the outer physical flesh. There is a strong link between illness and infirmity in the spirit and in the flesh and soul. We may be using terms with which some of you are not familiar. As we proceed through the book, we will make detailed descriptions of those terms which are likely to be in need of it. We want to encourage all readers to draw close to God (the God who authored the Bible) for the benefit of receiving His incredible love and His mercy. He is a true Father and will take care of those in need and is able to bring healing to both the spirit and the flesh. When one is in close proximity to Him, the healing power ends illness and heals emotional problems. He sees the beginning to the end of any problem we face and will give us His advice. Bruce one time was dealing with office workers who were at loggerheads and received the solution. Both Bruce and Alta Ada have been healed in the flesh by God several times and have seen friends healed from near terminal situations. God knows how to challenge one in order to develop the talents that He has given him. He knows just what is best for us. As Blaise Pascal, the famous 17th century mathematician and physicist, once said: "There is a God-shaped vacuum in the heart of every man which is never satisfied until it is filled with Jesus Christ." Micah 4:5 complements this statement: "For all people will walk every one in the name of his god, and we will walk in the name of the LORD our God for ever and ever." This Scripture shows that one does not have the option of whether to worship a god, but he will worship either the God of the Bible or one of his own making.

No person can ever be what he is called to be without coming into a deep relationship with God. Sadly, many people do not want to be in a relationship with Him. In order to help the reader, we need to lay down some foundational concepts. Unfortunately, the current Church in the West is very weak. (God Himself indicated this to us). There are a lot of reasons for this; and it does not mean that there are not some deep wells of spiritual water, but they are few and far between. Much of what we state is going to be relatively new for even those who have a strong background in various denominations. We have had to learn these things as the Holy Spirit has led us into some depths in the Scriptures. It is because of this that we use a lot of Scripture; and at times we give a superscript, with the passage indexed at the end of the chapter, or a direct quote. We need to build people up on a strong foundation—the Word of God. In doing this the reader will have an easier time establishing trust in God to move into some of the deeper understandings of what we call the spiritual realm, or spiritual universe. Becoming knowledgeable in God's Word will help to provide understanding of how, when, and why God heals.

Most people do not understand how God has made them and do not understand anything about their spirit. Until one goes through a second spiritual birth (most people do not), one cannot understand much of any helpful information about his spirit. Prior to going through a second birth our spirit is lifeless (cut off from the spiritual power of God's life-giving Spirit), and our flesh starts decaying even before birth and gradually becomes more degenerated by age and by diseases.

God is willing to give healing to illness in the flesh to any person who asks Him for it, believing in his heart that He will do so (it is this latter part that causes most requests to not be met). God demands of anyone seeking Him that he believes in his heart that He is. He will not likely heal someone who requests it with just an attitude that it is "worth a try." However, if one is thinking of asking God for healing, then he probably has belief in his heart; and God will more that meet him halfway. He is loving; kind; and, above all, merciful. He knows all that is in our hearts, and we do not.

Hebrews 11:6

[6] But without faith *it is* impossible to please *him*: for he that cometh to God must believe that he is, and *that* he is a rewarder of them that diligently seek him.

A problem is that if God were to give someone a healing of a problem just in the flesh, that person probably would not be able to maintain it for long if the spirit has not also been healed. If the person has a new spirit after going through the second birth, then he will have a much greater chance of maintaining the healing. Lasting healing in the flesh must be accompanied by healing of the spirit through the second birth and subsequent spiritual growth (not just intellectual growth). We see God using miracles of healing to draw people beyond healing of the physical problems into a spiritual renewal. This is one reason God uses healing— both in the past and in the present. The main reason God heals is because this is a significant part of who He is. It is so much a part of Him that people did not even have to do more than just touch Him in order to be healed. When one looks at those people the Lord Jesus Christ healed he can see that a large number turned and came to Him as their Lord and Savior. Some did not. He did not require it of those who did not want to come into a permanent relationship with him.

We will now start to look at some foundational concepts which are very important to understand if a person is seeking healing from God in both his spirit and his flesh. God is very much above all of us. We all can get more glimpses of Him from our experiences with Him. We should always be accurate and careful in interpretation of His Word pertaining to our experiences; but God is God, and we should never be dogmatic about what He will and will not do for any particular individual who seeks Him. He does not want anyone else to speak for another individual. All persons who have been born, and who will be in the future, have an equal chance with Him. He does not play favorites, and there are no barriers with Him for any person regardless of his past and background. He loves all and wishes all would choose to spend eternity with Him, but He has determined that will not occur without people seeking it His way, and we offer some glimpses later why this might be.

Foundational Concepts

Foundational concepts are just what the name indicates. Without placing these at the very foundation of our internal image of God's character and abilities, we might end up with a distorted view of God, the Bible, and the Creation. It would be like trying to solve a mathematical puzzle without knowing that one plus one is generally two. Placing these principles deeply into one's heart and mind is very important for his current and future decision making about plans for this phase of his eternal existence. We will give an overview in this chapter, and we will go into depth about some of these foundational concepts in subsequent chapters. When we use the name God, we are referring to the God who reveals Himself through the Scriptures in the Bible. He calls Himself by many names including the God of Abraham, Isaac, and Jacob; the God and Father of the Lord Jesus Christ; and He refers to Himself as the eternally existent one.

We can talk with God.

To understand anything about God, one has to study the Scriptures intensively. To understand any individual, one has to spend much time with that person. In the case of a historical person one has to read a lot of material about that person. When studying and learning about any individual, we have to be able to see through his eyes and to understand his mind and emotions. Translating this to the case of understanding God, one has to approach this by becoming God-centric instead of self-centric. One has to see what God wants, why He does what He does, and how He does what He does. The difference between God and a historical figure is that we can learn to ask Him questions readily and to get answers to those questions. This is not possible with a historical person. We can learn how to communicate back and forth with God using the methods He has revealed in the Scriptures.

God made this creation for His own eternal purposes.

Many people, when thinking of God and talking about Him, assume that He is like them.[1] In other words they look at God from a self-focused view and expect Him to fall into acting from the same set of motives which they use. People assume that God thinks like they do.[2] Few people think about God's feelings concerning an issue, nor would they consider that He is subject to emotions. While they assume that He is like them, they also seem to feel that He is distant, uninvolved, and impersonal. Few people make an effort to come into a relationship involving constant communication with God; and yet that is what He wishes to have with every single person who will ever live.[3]

God does not share all of His knowledge with men in this age.[4] He does get to know many people to some degree and a few people He knows very well. He gets to know only those who will let Him get to know them.[5] Most people do not want to have God know them because they understand at their deepest levels that they would have to make big changes in their plans and actions. When God speaks of knowing, we have to understand that He uses this word *knowing* in a much deeper sense than people usually do. God sees and hears everything about everyone who has ever lived. He sees and hears all of the thoughts and motivations for all actions that every single person has ever made or will ever make. When He uses the word *knowing*, He speaks of it as in a very close and intimate relationship. In this relationship there is discussion back and forth. Discussion with God is quite different in content from what one discusses with another person, but the principles for getting to know God well are the same as those for getting to know any person well. Each involves placing oneself in the shoes of the other—listening to him, understanding why he says what he says and does what he does, and seeing what he values and how he spends his time.

God adopts those who will let Him do so and brings them into His family.

God brings those people who seek His offer of adoption into His eternal family by a process similar to natural realm adoption and gives them a spiritual birth. When these people go through a spiritual birth, they get a new spirit residing in their spiritual heart (core). We will see that this spirit is an inner man with spiritual senses, and he has the ability to be in constant deep communication with God. Our inner man, if we will learn to listen to him, shares information and communications from God to us. We can learn how to operate in the spiritual realm as God teaches us through our spirit. Only God can teach an individual to operate in the spiritual realm. He becomes their spiritual father through adoption. In a process similar to how our natural parents trained us to know what our eyes were seeing[6] and what our ears were hearing in the natural realm, so God does for His children in the spiritual realm.

Sadly, most of God's children do not realize that they can work directly with God to learn how to operate in the spiritual realm. If they would learn from God, they would experience growth in their inner spirit man; and they would begin to mature in spiritual knowledge, strength, and power. None of this maturing can be brought about by those things we have learned as children, from school, or from college. Very little of it can come from any of our natural-life experiences.

The natural and the spiritual realms are approachable only through their own distinct set of six similar senses. If one has not been through the second birth, the only spiritual understanding he has is hearsay (or deceptions from demonic spirits). If one has been through the second birth but has never learned from God how to use his spiritual senses, then he is not much better off, despite his new birth, than one who has never been through it. There is a major exception to this. If God gives a second birth then that individual will spend eternity with Him even if he is not growing in this life.

God created two realms (universes) within the creation.

Later, we will learn more about the two universes in this creation. There is the natural universe (realm) made up of materials that can be seen, heard, touched, tasted, smelt, and arranged in space in a relationship to each other. This includes materials seen by an extension of our physical senses by devices such as telescopes and microscopes.

There is a spiritual universe (which may explain dark matter) which is somewhat parallel but is not able to be understood by natural senses and reasoning. All of the material we reason about, in either universe, is based on inputs from our senses which we arrange through our thought processes into an understanding of our environment. This spiritual realm is different enough to the natural realm in the laws by which it operates that our natural reasoning cannot comprehend it in any more than a distant, dim, and distorted way; and we also learn of it by hearsay. We emphasize that no amount of thinking with the natural mind and no amount of academic ability within the natural mind can comprehend anything of significance about this spiritual realm. The gap between the two realms is so great that it cannot be bridged without a person's gaining spiritual senses to inform his mind. It cannot be understood by natural man's reasoning and intellectual skills.[7] It has to be lived in and experienced within one's spirit. The only entrance for man into this spiritual realm is to go through a process of birth into this realm.[8] We shall discuss this "second" birth in detail later.

Man was created by God to be a spiritual being inside a body of flesh (natural materials). When man rebelled against God, he suffered death in his flesh; and his spirit was cut off from the spiritual energy and life which flowed into it from God so that in a manner it became a decaying remnant of what it had been. Man had been warned by God of the consequences of his rebellion in advance, and yet in the freedom to choose his own destiny mankind chose to listen to an evil spirit and in doing so allowed that evil spirit (the devil, Satan) to subject mankind in bondage to it (him).

The remnant spirit in men is able to function poorly, if at all, in being aware of the spiritual realm. This inner spiritual man we all have has lost almost all function in the analogous six senses that the natural flesh has.

It is very important to realize that while there are individual differences in the ability to interact with this spiritual realm, a person who has not been through the second birth has little more than a very rudimentary ability. Both God and (to a lesser extent) evil spirits can energize this dead spirit to some enhanced function temporarily. Evil spirits energize mediums on behalf of other souls enquiring, but these evil spirits do not tell the truth so there is little use to their advice.

The spiritual realm can only be understood by maturing spiritual realm senses.

People persist in thinking they can understand the spiritual realm with the use of natural realm knowledge and reasoning. There is insufficient knowledge to allow functioning of the natural realm mind in solving spiritual realm issues. However, the spiritual realm trained mind can solve natural realm situations. The laws which govern the spiritual realm are very different from those which describe the natural realm. The natural realm observations have led to the laws describing gravity and mechanics of various types, but these all breakdown when a powerful spirit being ma-

nipulates the natural realm. We will look at some of the miraculous events that God has performed later. These natural laws are
largely accurate; but none, including gravity, holds when power
from the spiritual realm is used. We see such power in walking on
water, being transported in the spirit, and other events. The spiritual materials are entirely different from the natural materials. The
only things in common are that both realms have laws and materials. To get some insight into these differences, one must think
about the power that the Lord Jesus Christ had over the natural
realm in all aspects of it. Consider the following miracles performed by the Lord Jesus Christ—turning water into wine, walking on water, healing people from many physical conditions and
illnesses, multiplying loaves and fish, calming a storm, and being
able to appear and disappear at His choosing (after His resurrection). Other miracles in Scripture include the physical transport-
ing of the evangelist Philip from one natural location to another
through spiritual power, resurrecting dead people, parting the Red
Sea, and assigning these powers to others (*e.g.*, Isaiah) for varied
lengths of time.

*The natural realm is in a state of death, cut off from the Life-
Giving Spirit of God.*

When Adam and Eve disobeyed God, they suffered the consequences about which God had forewarned them. Their spirits
were cut off from God's life-giving power, and their flesh was
subject to returning to dust. Spiritual death is defined as being
cut off from God. We should also understand that when man died
a spiritual death, God subjected the rest of the natural realm to a
spiritual death.[9] Both man and the natural realm are now under
judgment, and both the flesh of man and the natural realm will
be replaced and done away with in the future. The reality of this
death is that even though the natural realm looks fine to us, in
fact it is virtually lifeless compared to the spiritual realm. One
could conceptualize that it is in an advanced state of *rigor mortis*. In reading Psalm 29 one will see the description of various
geographic features responding to the voice of God. This psalm

and similar passages in other places, suggest that there is a natural-realm representation of everything in the spiritual realm.[10] An important Scripture in this respect is 2 Kings 6. The spiritual part can still respond to the awesome power in God; but the natural part, being dead, responds less well, if at all. The Lord describes what occurs in the spiritual realm in order to let us see the difference between what we have in death and what we can have in gaining spiritual life through the second birth. One must keep this concept in mind when describing natural laws, such as gravity; for such laws hold only over a narrow range of space and time; and then they only hold most of the time but break down when the natural realm is subject to a spiritual power.

Forecasting and prophecy and the passage of time

God has power over time. The very concept of time is not the same in the spiritual realm as it is in the natural realm. We need to understand that time in the natural realm does not change at the same rate as in the spiritual realm. For example, in the book of Revelation the Apostle John sees the birth of the Lord Jesus in the spiritual realm after it had occurred in the natural realm. In addition, we are told in other Scripture that the Lord Jesus was slain before the foundation of the Earth.

One has to undergo training and learning in the spiritual realm to appreciate just how the two realms interrelate. We could come up with various theories to explain the above observations of Scripture, but there is a better way to find out and that is to ask God to teach us.

In fact, the passage of time between these realms does not appear to be parallel. God can see ahead of an event which will occur in the natural realm and know what the outcomes will be. For example, the Lord Jesus knew and stated that, if the people of Sodom and Gomorrah (which were destroyed by God due to the amount of sin within them) had known as much about Him as the cities of Tyre and Sidon knew, these two cities would have repented of their sin and would not have been destroyed. As we think about this and similar statements, we can see that God knew what over-all historical development He wanted in the creation that He was about to make. He decided on the details of this creation that He made ahead of time in order to fulfill His purposes for it. His final purposes will be fulfilled in this creation in the manner described in the book of Revelation. This is a book which foretells the final judgments of God on this creation and then describes the beginnings of the next age. God knows the details of all people who will ever exist to the extent of knowing how many hairs are on their heads and of knowing all of the thoughts they have ever had and the motivations for all of their actions.

Are people responsible for their thoughts and actions?

God holds all people responsible for the thoughts they persist in working with and the actions they take at every single moment in time. There is no escaping God's notice in any detail of one's life. People can choose to not believe in Him but He has stated centuries ago in written format (Romans 1) that all people have knowledge of Him through observing the creation. There will be no excuse for those who willfully despise the reconciliation that God has offered to them. He considers this reconciliation to have been purchased at great cost to Him, and no one will have any excuse when standing before Him at the final judgment when He will be seated on a great white throne. People will spend the rest of the ages to come (an eternity) either living with Him or separated forever from Him. This raises the obvious question as to which choice would be better.

Is it better to spend eternity with God?

To answer this question one should turn to look at what things he would desire to be present in an eternity of time. Would one wish to be perpetually filled with a sense of great joy, great peace, of being intensely loved and desired, and of feeling fulfillment in all aspects of one's life? Would he pay a price in this life to have a future of peace and harmony with all of his fellow people?

Does one desire patience from others?

Does one desire others to be willing to bear with us as we struggle with issues while we learn?

Does one appreciate others always being honest with us and never deceiving us?

Does one want full knowledge of his circumstances?

Does one want glorious incredible light (as opposed to unending darkness)?

Does one wish for an environment where he can be creative and valued for his unique contributions, never being slighted or made to feel inadequate?

Does one value a sense of excitement about the future?

Does one wish to spend his time surrounded by great beauty and continuous innovation?

If the answer to any of these and many similar questions is yes, then he will want to spend eternity with God in His Kingdom.

What will it be like in an eternity separated from God?

Although God is longsuffering, patient with people, kind, and compassionate, He also is true to His Word. After exhausting all possibilities of reconciling a person to Him, He will judge that individual who refuses to accept His salvation offered in the Lord Jesus Christ. One of the seven Spirits of God is the Spirit of Judgment and Burning (Isaiah 4:4). Another one of the Spirits, by contrast, is the Spirit of Grace and Supplications (Zechariah 12:10). It is this Spirit which is linked with His longsuffering, gentleness, and kindness. The seven spirits are a fundamental part of God's character. Those who refuse to reconcile to God will be faced with coming under the Spirit of Judgment and Burning. This judgment is much delayed by His other character traits of longsuffering, gentleness, and kindness. God's character is expressed through all of His Spirits. People are made in His Image and also express one of their many spirits in various situations.

Those people who come under the spirit of judgment and burning will have some dwelling; they may be able to visit back and forth (Luke 16:9); and there will be degrees of punishment based on their works in their life in the natural realm (Revelation 20:12). There will be a purifying fire that will burn continuously; but it will not consume anything, for God will use this to keep the souls and spirits in a situation where the fire purifies the eternal abode so that there will not exist in the ages to come a place which is impure. Relationships will not be satisfying; truth will not be valued; deceit will be common; there will be tears and remorse which cannot be stemmed and will never come to an end. There will be no feeling of fulfillment. There will be no hope of a brighter tomorrow. There will be little of beauty. There will be darkness such as was seen at the time of the plagues of Egypt. There will be no real love or admiration. There will be no patience or understanding.

Is God really going to condemn someone He made to such a grim future? What kind of God would do that?

This is a commonly-used ploy people make for not wanting to deal with God and face the changes this would cause them to have to make in their lives.

God has written about these two different futures we mentioned above. God is committed to truth and will never lie. He is going to keep His integrity and truthfulness in spite of all of these excuses. That is what they are, for God offers multiple opportunities for each person to reconcile with Him until such a point where He can see that it is futile. We all know the consequences of not dealing with God, for He has made this very clear to each of us.

At the final great white throne judgment one will be judged on whether he has accepted the sacrifice of the Lord Jesus Christ for his sins and submitted to Him as his Lord. If he has, he will spend eternity with God. If he has not he will spend eternity in some degree of continual punishment and will always be separated from God. God has a value system which is quite different from fallen man's (we are all fallen unless we go through the second birth), and He is looking for people to spend eternity with Him who esteem His values. These people will be important for God's plan in the future ages. These values include being at peace, being joyful, being loving, valuing truth above all else, being self-sacrificing, being patient, and being willing to be longsuffering to obtain a greater future good. These people desire to serve rather than rule over others. The future ages, which God has ordered, will depend on having people with such character traits as detailed above. These people will be unified in spirit (team players).

Those people condemned to eternal separation from God were never willing to invest in these qualities, and they wanted their rewards from other men. They were not prepared to allow themselves to be trained for a future where they would not be in charge. God is so far above individual people in His intellect, skills, and power that there is no point for Him to have His entire plans changed for self-focused individuals. Such people would cause disruption in the ages to come if allowed to be present with God, and it would also be unfair to those who followed God. To dwell with God in eternity, one must develop a core attitude of being a servant to his fellows; and he must be able to live in peace with and in harmony of spirit with those who share this life with God and with him.

Those who choose to live with God will not have to meet any quotas. They have to accept the Lord Jesus Christ as Savior and submit to His call on their life as Lord. His yoke is easy and not burdensome. People will be there from all races and nations. There is, so to speak, equal opportunity. If anything, the people who make this choice are the less successful in worldly wealth and wisdom (1 Corinthians 1:26-27). They are not the proud people but rather are contrite and humble. God hates pride, for it raises a person in his own esteem to the point in which he does not feel a need for God.

The Bible

People react to the Bible with a wide array of emotions and understanding. The Bible was written by God through His influencing many men. He did not dictate it, but He did safeguard the truth in it. It is put together in such a way that foundational messages from the entire Scripture are built from many people writing centuries apart. These people may not have seen how their part would interface with a different part.

It is historical in that it details the way God has related to mankind through the ages. It is very relevant to every age and people, since it details how to come into a relationship with God and the desirability of this.

It provides a description of the anatomy of and the workings of the spiritual man. The spiritual man is the inner spirit. The Scriptures show how this inner man relates to the physical flesh. It gives information for how this inner man can be strengthened and how he can mature.

The Bible reveals what is going on in this current age.

The Bible gives future plans of God for mankind. It gives information about the relationship God expects to have with men.

We also learn in it that God has put the Bible text together in such a way that a lot is hidden and must be diligently searched out.

It is also written in such a way that it is living. The fact that it is living allows it to interact intelligently with the reader. This is not a novel thing, and it is not unique to the Bible; but in the Bible the life is much more powerful and pervasive than that in any other other writing.

Consider that, when a person writes a book he will target certain audiences; and these people will respond to the material in a a variety of ways. This is living but is very limited in power in comparison to that in the Bible. God in His infinite knowledge and wisdom wrote the Scriptures so that every person has a personalized message which it conveys to him. It is an answer to all of one's questions about himself and his environment. This individual message does require seeking out.

Hebrews 11:6

[6] But without faith *it is* impossible to please *him*: for he that cometh to God must believe that he is, and *that* he is a rewarder of them that diligently seek him.

Every person who is born into this world comes into it with the expectation of God for a unique contribution that he can make for now and for eternity. Most choose to not take up their unique destiny. That is their choice, and it is not God's choice. He will never compel. He will never manipulate. He is always considerate, concerned, and caring. He knows each person far better than that individual knows himself.

The Current Age in which we live

God chose to make this creation and this age in it in such a way that He could acquire a family of spiritual children who will have been trained to function so they can rule and reign with God in the ages to come. This requires character features which God foresaw. He chose for His creation this history which is currently playing out.

He created angels, who are spiritual beings like Himself. He created men, a hybrid of spirit and of "natural" materials. He gave each of these classes (angels and men) a choice to voluntarily come under His guidance in a loving relationship, looking to Him to provide leadership and direction in all things. These would spend eternity with God and would share in future ages in His future plans. The men would be His children, and the angels would be His ministers.

Both men and angels are able to make a choice free of any manipulation or coercion about where they wish to spend eternity. There are only two choices– for God or against Him.

As time goes by, those angels and men who reject God come to hold less of His image within themselves; and they acquire the character of antagonists to the character of God, since His image is no longer seen in them. Men take on the character of the fallen angels. There is no truth present; there is no love present. There is no hope present.

Satan was the first angel to fall from a relationship with God and now opposes everything of God. He successfully tempted Adam and Eve to follow him and in doing so gained a God-given legal right to rule over the earth in this age. Before Adam and Eve fell, they had the right to rule over the earth.

Those people who reconcile to God and are adopted back into His family have power delegated to them to work with God to take back the works of the devil.

The character of the devil is such that he and his evil angels (demons) act only to steal, kill, and destroy mankind and the creation. Satan has the title "father of lies," and there is no truth in him. Men are born under the image of the devil, but they do know the difference between good and evil. Until a man goes through the second birth, he cannot escape the character in which he was born. The power of the flesh to do evil (God counts pride as one of the most evil things) is very powerful, and only God can overcome it when he gives a second birth to those people who see the evil of this age and want to escape it. Evil may not appear as such to us; in fact many people appear to do good and kind things. It is only after escaping from the clutches of the devil and spending time being trained by God in the spiritual realm that one can see the whole truth of God's view that all man does is evil. We can see it in the natural state we are in also, since we retain the ability to know the difference between good and evil.

God continues to limit the devil, as seen in Job 1. God does this in all aspects of the creation so that today we do not see the complete revelation of pure evil, but we can see many attributes of it.

In the creation we can all still discern the nature and character of God (Romans 1)

Through the last 7000 years of the creation Satan has developed a highly-honed propaganda machine to smear and demean the character of God and to appeal to the flesh of mankind. With these approaches he is able to destroy many souls and subject them to an eternity spent apart from God. He hates God, and he hates the image of God seen in collective humanity. Leading up to the crucifixion of the Lord Jesus Christ the devil had Him beaten to where His face was unrecognizable.

Isaiah 52:14

[14] As many were astonied at thee; his visage was so marred more than any man, and his form more than the sons of men:

The devil in these days has destroyed, as best he is able, the image of God in mankind. He will never completely succeed in this because God will not allow that. He mars man with disease, infirmity, addiction, cruelty to one another, and many other similar negative things.

There are other Gods

Throughout the natural realm history people have worshiped various deities. God made man in such a manner that he has to worship something (see Micah 4:5 quoted above).

Many worship such items such as power, fame, prestige, and money.

God states in the Scriptures (John 17:3) that He is the only true

God. Then who are these other deities, and how does one decide which God is the true God? In deciding who is the true God we see God (who wrote the Bible) defeat many other deities—including the gods of Pharaoh, the god Baal, and many of the gods of the people who occupied the Promised Land prior to God's giving it to Israel. Therefore power is one way of discerning who is the true God and this victory goes to the God Who wrote the Bible. He describes Himself with many names and we have mentioned several above. He is the God of Abraham, Isaac, and Jacob. He is the God and Father of the Lord Jesus Christ. He is the eternally existent One.

In the passage of time God has allowed Bruce to see two other deities; both were evil spirits. One was an Egyptian God and the other a Goddess of Hate (Styx)—an ancient River God. In each occurrence Bruce felt the emotional force of waves of hatred coming from each. These gods can place a mantle of hate on whomever they choose to influence. These gods are high-level demons. The hate is felt as a strong force. It has a considerable power to it and would be compelling to many people who had no idea of the source of the hate they might be feeling. Such spirits would place a mantle of hate over a person and try to have him associate it with some object, situation, or another person or group of people. That is why we will discuss taking all of our emotions and thoughts captive so we can try to discern the source of the thoughts and emotions we are experiencing. No one would want to act under such a spirit if he knew what was happening, but he cannot know that without his spiritual vision being developed. This development comes only after the second birth.

God can cast spirits over large geographic areas and over nations. These influence the entire population, such as the spirit of slumber over Israel (Romans 11:8). Higher-level evil spirits can also do similar things but with less power and with less influence than God.

God states that wisdom is justified by her children (Matthew

11:19). Thus, the followers of a deity will behave like that deity. If one wants to know the character of any other god, look at the beliefs, attitudes, and acts of the followers of that god.

At the very foundation all of these evil deities are revealed to hate the true God and His children, as do the followers of these deities. These evil deities will frequently emanate a powerful force of hate.

Bruce can contrast this to the powerful force of love emanating from the true God. This force of love from God is directed generally to all people but can be increased in power to those people for whom God wishes to do this.

Therefore, the motivations and emotions of the followers of any deity reveal the character of that god. No other god than the true God can love. There will be lusts, envy, and jealousy; but no other god can produce a spiritual force of love. This is why the Bible majors on being able to tell the true followers of the true God by their spirit of love (it is a force and results in actions). There are many false followers, planted by the devil—described as tares. These do not have a spirit of love.

Can other gods heal?

To receive spiritual and physical healing or just physical healing, one has to deal with the true God. Any other god may appear to give healing; but it will be of less power than the true God gives, and it always comes with a blood commitment or an oath of allegiance which impacts future generations. The true God will never do this. He heals freely and out of compassion, not for control. Any spirit of control is always evil. We are discussing some of these foundations so that the reader can understand all of the issues pertaining to healing. At the end of this chapter we will discuss precautions to take when one is seeking divine healing. One needs to be aware of and cautious with snares and traps when seeking healing.

A few important observations

The Character of God and of the devil

God is truth and light (in both the spiritual realm and natural realm).

The devil exudes lies and darkness (spiritual realm), but in the natural realm he can appear deceptively as an angel of light.

God's truth is critically important for maintaining the fabric of a society. When we downgrade it, we sin against God.

Spiritual beings are superior to natural beings.

Angels were created with more spiritual power than man and with more complete knowledge of the spiritual realm than fallen man. Adam and Eve had spiritual knowledge which was corrupted at the fall from grace in the Garden of Eden.

What sin is

Sin is the act(s) of being disobedient to God's stated and implied standards. One can sin without ever having consciously expressed those standards because God placed these standards in the minds and consciences of men. Sin is not limited to overt actions and includes thought patterns which violate God's standards. The tendency to sin arises in three broad categories:

1. The lust of the flesh which is allowing impulses of the flesh to dictate our behavior (we will look at this further in Chapter 7)

2. The lust of the eyes which entices us to modify our behavior in order to covet those things in our environment which look appealing

3. The pride of life which is self-confidence based within our own natural abilities which entices us to act indepen-

dently of God and which leads to our ultimate downfall into eternity without God unless we repent of this strong driving force

The demonic powers are well aware of how to promote these three categories of sin in each of our lives and do so by speaking to our spirit and to our flesh. We will look at spiritual communication later. They are far more intelligent and subtle than man and readily deceive many (in fact the vast majority of people). These people allow themselves to be deceived initially, but after a while they become insensitive to their situation.

The World System

There is a world system which Satan heads and which provides false education, false philosophies, and false knowledge about every aspect of the creation. There is distortion in every area. Truth is present in the natural realm only where the work of God is going on and where God is present. Men can deceive. Spiritual beings can deceive only as they act through men. Truth is always present in the spiritual realm, and it is only as we learn after the second birth to operate in this realm that we can operate consistently in truth. The Scripture below is an eternal truth.

Luke 6:43

[43] For a good tree bringeth not forth corrupt fruit; neither doth a corrupt tree bring forth good fruit.

In the natural realm a corrupt man may hide his intentions from another person, but those who can discern the spirit of the man will not be deceived.

There is still enough of God's presence and truth seen in the creation for any man who chooses to do so to come into relationship with God. No one has anyone to blame except himself for his final judgment before the great white throne.

Summary

These foundational points give us a start to understanding our current age and the situation into which we have been born. We have looked at some of the issues and we will elaborate on many of them in more detail. The reader may ask why we are going into this detail if he just wants a sore leg to be healed, for example. The reason is that we are as much concerned with spiritual healing as we are with natural healing of the flesh. Spiritual healing comes only as one gets into the right relationship with God, his Creator. Without this relationship being fixed no physical healing can withstand the assaults of the evil spirits. Because they do not understand how these spirits work, many people have had a healing stolen by the evil spirits confusing them with false physical symptoms. As one has his spirit filled with the love and power of God, he can expect complete physical healing if he is able to bless God (Psalm 103:1-5). Blessing God is a high mark, and probably few achieve it. One cannot promise how God will behave toward anyone else or even toward himself, since none of us knows the depths of our own heart.

We begin in the next chapter discussing the imperative to have the correct order in our minds of the relationship of the spiritual realm and the natural realm for getting our information and knowledge in any and in all situations in which we find ourselves.

As we go further, the book will become more focused on helping those who are close to going through the second birth and those who have gone through it. However, seeing the logical explanations of the spiritual realm will be of interest to any reader. Keep in mind that the natural man (either one who has not undergone the second birth or has not matured after it) cannot discern the truth of spiritual material. He has to accept or reject it based on hearsay evidence.

Precautions about seeking divine healing

No one, and the authors are no exception, can be absolutely sure that God will choose to heal a particular person from a particular health issue. Bruce has seen several people through the years in his medical practice that had been to a healing service and told him they had been healed. In few cases was this true. One woman with diabetes who claimed healing stopped taking insulin, came back two years later with uncontrolled diabetes, and lost a leg from gangrene. Bruce had asked her to follow up closely and had told her at the time that, if she had been healed, the lab tests would indicate it. She did not follow up and did not take the lab tests.

There are various situations where one may seek healing—people with pain, people with various chronic illnesses, people with cancer, and people with life-threatening circumstances. We strongly suggest that any individual seeking God's healing let his physician know what he is doing and ask his physician to monitor him for results. When God heals an illness in the flesh it will be apparent to both the patient and the physician. It does not hurt to do this even if one has experienced God's healing previously. Doing so helps a person to receive definite feedback that is positive or alerts a person to the fact that he needs to explore why God is choosing to not heal him at this time. It also serves to ease the concerns of the physician; and when someone receives this healing, then God will get the glory.

The question arises about continuing medical treatment while waiting for God to heal him. A person has to work with God and with his physician on this issue and come to a point of peace in his soul. If someone in faith wants to stop a vital medication then he should be monitored more closely by his doctor. A person would need to hear very clearly from God that this is the path to follow. Faith will be discussed later, but for now we need to understand that faith is more than a hope. Faith actually comes only when one knows that God has spoken to him and has no doubt in the matter. Only a person who has learned through many experiences to know the voice of God and His many ways of speaking to him in various circumstances should attempt something that could be life threatening. Even then, a safety plan with the physician is wise. If one has any doubt that God has said that He would heal him, then let the doctor treat him. God is not offended by this and in fact the Scriptures mandate it. We will discuss the issue of never walking beyond one's faith later. It is akin to leaping off the pinnacle of the temple, a temptation from Satan that the Lord Jesus Christ did not take.

Pride is a frequent cause of falsely thinking that God has spoken healing to an individual. Demons can be great mimics, and a person needs spiritual discernment. We would suggest never trusting an intermediary who tells one that God is going to heal him. Prophets are not without error; and where there is a life-threatening issue then one can confidently deal directly only with God.

In our experience God always lets us know that He is going to heal. In 2010 Bruce had the elders pray over him for healing of an inflammatory generalized arthritis. About three nights later the Holy Spirit said quite clearly, "I am going to cool your joints, and your healing has commenced." Bruce had no doubt that he would be healed because there was no doubt this was God's letting him know. Incidentally, no physician would have expressed this the way that the Lord God did.

In addition, Bruce had an ulcer on his lower left eyelid, diagnosed by an optometrist as a basal cell cancer in 2002. It seemed to Bruce that the devil was trying to "get in his face" over a recent success. God spoke to Bruce and told him not to worry, that the lesion would dry up and drop off. About three weeks later while at a church service on Cape Cod the pastor, who had a prophetic gifting, said to Bruce, without knowing about the situation: "That thing is going to dry up and drop off." This confirmed the Scripture in 2 Corinthians 13:1 that a word is established in the mouth of two or three witnesses. The lesion left unnoticed by Bruce.

Usually, God is quite clear about a matter. If there is doubt, then one should not presume God will heal him because it indicates that one is not sure God has spoken to him. God does not hide His light under a bushel.

No one can ever give another person a 100% rule about God. If he could, then he would know more about the situation than God. In healing one can get advice about the process from others; but ultimately he has to deal with God, the healer. Alta Ada addressed being healed by those with gifts of healing in her book *Healing: What God has Provided for His Children* so we will not discuss that in this book.

We have been healed many times of non urgent matters. One night having been scheduled to fly from Seattle to New Orleans the following day in December 2015, we both started developing severe 'flu like symptoms. We had understood that God wanted us to make the trip. Therefore, we asked Him to heal us. Both of us awoke the next morning quite well and made the trip uneventfully. This was not a life-threatening situation. We are aware of God's helping people with postoperative pain. He knows better how to help with such a situation than anyone else.

It is always well worth seeking healing from God because His healings are perfect, as we will discuss later. Those of physicians are frequently partial, at best, and can have potential side effects. There have been times in our lives when God has said to wait. There are frequently timing issues, as we see in the Scriptures. God is in control of these timing issues. It is all right to keep reminding God that one wants healing, but one should always respectfully defer the decision to the will of God. If we do not defer to Him, it is possible that He will give us what we want; but it may well damage the future relationship with Him (Psalm 106:15).

Healing of the Church

God spoke to Bruce one evening at a prayer service for breaking a drought in 1998. He stated that the churches are weak. He indicated that He wanted us to teach His people in order to strengthen them. Spiritual weakness in the Church is an illness. When we use the term Church with a capital letter, we are speaking of the true members of the body of the Lord Jesus Christ, who are those to whom God has given the second birth. In the spiritual realm illness is due to a loss or a weakening of God's relationship with a person with resulting weakness in spiritual strength, spiritual wisdom, spiritual understanding, and spiritual knowledge. This has certainly occurred and persists in the Church in the West. We will discuss this further in later chapters. When a spiritual illness occurs there is always an accompanying illness in the flesh; and this is seen in the members of the Church. These members, in general, have a distorted and weak relationship with the Lord Jesus Christ, who is the head of the Church.

Superscript References for this Chapter

1. Psalm 50:21

2. Isaiah 55:8-9

3. Matthew 10:32, 1 Thessalonians 5:17, and Revelation 22:17

4. Deuteronomy 29:29

5. Matthew 7:22-23

6. 2 Kings 6:15-18

7. 1 Corinthians 2, especially verse 14

8. John 3:1-12, especially vs. 11, 13-16

9. Romans 8:18-22

10. Exodus 25:40

How we can Bless God and Receive Healing

Chapter 2

We want to make it clearly understood at the outset that God heals people without their being in a deep relationship with Him. Sometimes He heals those in no relationship with Him. The authors have each been healed early on in their understanding of the Lord God and His Kingdom. Neither of us had anywhere near the knowledge and understanding that the Holy Spirit has since given us. Our earlier book, *Healing*, by Alta Ada Williams, discusses many Scriptures pertaining to healing.

Bruce was healed three times from chronic arthritis. The first time was after God initiated his interest in healing and led him to have the elders lay hands on him for healing (see James 5). This occurred in a church that had a positive doctrinal statement about healing; but in the laying on of the hands the pastor said, in similar words, that this might or might not work. In spite of that statement Bruce had been faithful to perform what the Holy Spirit was speaking to him; and two weeks later a very severe, painful, chronically inflamed ankle joint was healed spontaneously. On the second occasion the healing was by a declaration of a prophet. The third time the elders did believe when they laid hands on Bruce. This was the occasion when the Holy Spirit spoke to Bruce three nights later and said, "Your joints are being cooled and your healing has begun." Deformities were allowed to persist; but the inflammation is no longer present, and pain is minimal. The reasons for needing three healings are too complex to go into in this account.

One can ask why one will benefit from a close relationship with Him, since God heals people regardless of their relationship with Him and their knowledge of His character. There are several reasons why one should get into a close relationship with God and subsequently become mature in his spirit. God generally defers to His people about the intensity of the relationship they develop with Him (James 4:8). We will discuss the reasons for the need of the close relationship now.

It is highly desirable to be in a close relationship with God for healing.

1. There are promises to heal all diseases (Psalm 103:1-5) when one blesses God. To bless God, one have to be in a very mature relationship with Him. This does not mean that He will not heal all disease for someone who is not in a mature relationship with Him; He does what He feels is needed for every person, and there are no 100% rules about what God will do. He sees the depths of the heart of each of us in a way which we cannot. He also keeps His own counsel. When one reviews all of the miracles the Lord Jesus Christ did during His advent, many were specific for a particular condition; and a small number were such that all of the diseases were healed. Therefore, it is desirable to be able to bless the Lord and have all diseases healed.

2. When one is in a close relationship with God, he will have learned how to stand against and resist the devil. He needs to do this because the devil focuses on destroying healings that are performed by God. If Satan can get a person to believe that he was not healed or that the condition has returned, then God is discredited. Bruce noted in his healings that the demonic spirits were persistent in trying to induce similar symptoms to those he had; he needed to understand this and resist it. Without understanding how spiritual man is put together and works, one can fail to mature and to resist the evil spirits. One develops residing strength in his spirit only through a close and a mature relationship with God. Our earlier books, both *How to be Led by the Spirit of God: Maturing in the Spirit* and *Spirit* both discuss in great detail the anatomy and workings of spiritual man. We need to note and understand that our

natural body of flesh was designed to support the spiritual man, not the other way around.

3. It is only when a person gets a new spirit that he can resist the devil and maintain a healing. This means becoming an adopted child of God. He will only adopt those who place their trust in the salvation He offers by accepting the sacrifice of the Lord Jesus Christ on the cross as a substitute for his own sins and accepting Him also as His Lord and Savior. In addition, he must confess that the Lord Jesus Christ is his Lord and Savior before men; and he must seek direction from Him for all decision making, since He is his Lord. Many think they have been through the second birth and have not. Contemplate the Scripture below and make sure that you have done the above and that you are in submission to God in all things.

Matthew 7:22–24

[22] Many will say to me in that day, Lord, Lord, have we not prophesied in thy name? and in thy name have cast out devils? and in thy name done many wonderful works? [23] And then will I profess unto them, I never knew you: depart from me, ye that work iniquity. [24] Therefore whosoever heareth these sayings of mine, and doeth them, I will liken him unto a wise man, which built his house upon a rock.

It is so difficult for people outside the true faith to understand the Christian faith because there are many tares among the true wheat. These tares sound very like, and look very like, the wheat. The Lord states that He is leaving these tares in place until the end of this age.

4. A person is completely healed of all diseases of the flesh only after the second birth. In addition there must be continuing maturing of the inner man. Without maturing in one's spirit, a person has spiritual malnourishment and will not have the spiritual strength to make the flesh sub-

mit to his inner man. This is similar to the medical condition of Failure to Thrive. A person with a weak spirit may
not be much better off in the natural realm phase of life
than someone who has not been through the second birth,
except he does have eternal salvation.

Therefore, in the rest of this book we are going to discuss the issues one needs to understand to position him for having healing
of all of his diseases. This requires having received the second
birth and then maturing in the inner man. We will talk about how
to needed to undergo maturing. In the rest of this chapter we will
address some general issues for all who wish to ask God for healing and how they can be in a position to be likely to receive it.

The Church will be healed as leaders and members become individually spiritually strengthened by coming into the relationship
with God where He is their head in all decisions that affect His
Kingdom. There are Scriptures pertaining to what this does not
involve. An example is that the types of food one eats would not
be an issue but; if eating a certain food harms the conscience of a
weaker brother it would be an issue. The Kingdom of Heaven is
very much concerned about our relationship with God and with
our brethren in the Church.

General Thoughts about asking God for healing

When it comes to asking God the Father for healing through the
name of His Son, the Lord Jesus Christ, one is approaching a
Holy God personally through the name of His Son—the Lord Jesus Christ (the only legal basis we have for any request of God
the Father). God tells us to ask, seek, and knock when making any
request; and there is a degree to which one must persist. He wants
people to seek Him diligently. We must be aware that when *name*
is used in Scripture, it represents character.

The bases of all of the healings described in the Scripture and
performed by the Lord Jesus Christ are faith in God (faith in His
whole character is preferred but sometimes people may have faith

just for healing); and belief in the heart of His ability and willingness to heal. The largest stumbling block to receiving divine healing is the lack of a firm belief in the spiritual heart that God is willing to heal; and to heal at the time requested. Acquiring any belief in the heart, as opposed to the mind, making a transient assent is a much more prolonged process and is nothing like having just an intellectual agreement that God will heal (which is more like a hope). It is very important for people to study the Scriptures and let God show them what faith, hope, and belief are and what they are not. There are great promises in Mark 11:23-24 for what a person can perform and request which are related to the beliefs which reside in the structures of the spiritual heart. We will talk further later in this book about acquiring belief in the heart and acquiring faith; and we will discuss what hope is. God tells us that without faith it is impossible to please Him, and so no one can be in a position to bless God without faith and belief in the heart.

Hebrews 11:6

⁶ But without faith *it is* impossible to please *him*: for he that cometh to God must believe that he is, and *that* he is a rewarder of them that diligently seek him.

God is very kind and merciful, and He makes His own decisions about when He will heal. There are many issues which may be present in one's life which may cause God to say, "No" until they are remedied. In the Kingdom of Heaven there are no rules pertaining to what one can and cannot do. God's personality (character) is such that he is drawn to people with need and with a broken contrite spirit and heart. The Kingdom of Heaven is built on peace, joy, and righteousness. It exudes love and loving kindness. There is unity of all the spirits of people. It may surprise people, even in the Church, that there are no behavioral rules in heaven. It is the Spirit, and His character, which holds all things in order. The Apostle Paul states:

1 Corinthians 10:23

²³ All things are lawful for me, but all things are not expedient: all things are lawful for me, but all things edify not.

We are not sure why this is so, since there are clearly laws in heaven for the functioning of the spiritual realm structures, such as the designs of the temple shown to Moses. There are rules about demonic spirits being confined to the earth. There is a hierarchical order in the Kingdom of Heaven. It seems that there is no need for behavioral rules in heaven. We surmise that there is no need for such rules because there is no evil in Heaven. All spirits are perfected in the positive emotions of love, joy, and peace—so there should not be any frictions between spirits. Evil spirits, when present, always have contention between spirits; and this always occurs with the negative emotions such as pride (which is the basis for all disagreement), anger, jealousy, and hate (Proverbs 13:10).

Whenever anyone expresses these negative emotions, he is not in a mode of trying to bring people together in a perfect bond. Fear may make people seem to come together; but it really does not do so in the heart, although it may compel behavior. We further surmise that God insists on His people in the eternal kingdom having positive emotions (see Scripture below). This is a key requirement for God. Those who have not been through the second birth are for eternity subject to the negative emotions, and will never experience true peace, joy, or love. As an aside, it would be very interesting to do a study about the impact of the general expressions of love and charitable caring within a society over time and graph it against the number of behavioral rules in a society.

1 John 4:18

²⁸ There is no fear in love; but perfect love casteth out fear: because fear hath torment. He that feareth is not made perfect in love.

God looks at the content of one's spiritual heart and, to some extent, the mind to decide how He is going to respond to various requests from that person who petitions Him. The Scripture tells us that only God (not even that individual) knows the entire content of a man's heart. God looks at an individual by examing the content of the spiritual heart.

Proverbs 27:19

[19] As in water face *answereth* to face, so the heart of man to man.

Few people are healed by God today.

One sees few healings by God. He does not heal through a physician or through the medical system, but rather He heals directly. There are no surgical wounds or drug side effects. Sometimes the healing is instantaneous, and sometimes it is not.

God does not oppose going to a physician, but His healing is far superior. There are a lot of issues in this world which are not really eternal issues in the Kingdom of God. The Apostle Paul writes about them in 1 Corinthians 8:1-13. The conscience is reset constantly as one gains greater understanding and knowledge of the Kingdom of Heaven. We believe seeking healing through the medical system is not a sin for some; but it is sternly rebuked by and punished by God as one has more authority, spiritual maturity, and spiritual strength. Read the account of King Asa below.

2 Chronicles 16:12

[12] And Asa in the thirty and ninth year of his reign was diseased in his feet, until his disease *was* exceeding *great*: yet in his disease he sought not to the LORD, but to the physicians.

The role of faith in healing

Romans 14:23

[23] And he that doubteth is damned if he eat, because *he eateth* not of faith: for whatsoever *is* not of faith is sin.

It is important to God that we do not walk beyond our faith. Many people act as if faith is a blind belief or hope; it is not, and we will explain what it is later. God regards doing this as sin because we are doing these acts by the will of the flesh and not by the will of God. God judged the flesh as sinful in the Garden of Eden, and it has its own will (John 1:13).

When we do these acts by the will of the flesh, then we get into an area where we just hope that God will do something. One has to be certain that God will heal him before deciding not to seek medical attention. To be certain of God's healing him, a person must know through learning how to be sure whether God, an evil spirit, or even his own wicked flesh is communicating with him. To do something without faith is the sin that the devil tried to make the Lord Jesus Christ commit in tempting Him to jump off of the pinnacle of the Temple.

One should never rely on another spirit to tell him what God will do. God forbids any spirit intermediaries in a relationship with Him. God does sometimes use a prophetic voice to let a person know about healing as He did with the ancient kings' seeking wisdom from Elijah and Elisha. He does not someone praying to any spirit other than Him.

It is always reasonable to seek the guidance of a true prophet regarding being healed by God, and God blesses that; but unless one has discernment in the spiritual realm (few do), then he may not know if he is dealing with a true prophet (many are not). It is better and safer always to deal with God directly and let the prophetic people give exhortation, edification, and comfort (encouragement) (1 Corinthians 14:3).

Of the issues we dealt with in the book *Healing* regarding why healings do not occur we noted that one of the major issues is a self-limitation God places on Himself in geographic areas where there is wide-spread unbelief in the things of God (Matthew 13:58). We will discuss these issues no further for now since this book is concerned about spiritual and physical healing upon which one can depend upon and which are mentioned in Psalm 103:1-5.

Promises of Healing we can be certain of when we make the effort

When God conveys something in written or spoken form, one can depend on His being faithful to fulfill those words. Truth and keeping truth are the most foundational parts of God's complex character (Psalm 138:2). He will place all other issues under these. Nearly all the promises of God are conditional. That is, a man (or men) must perform some requirements to obtain the promise. Therefore, if we can ascertain exactly what blesses God, we can be certain to experience the healing of physical illnesses, infirmities, and other health problems described in Psalm 103:1-5. The condition to receiving this is that we are a blessing to God (based on His definition of blessing). Getting healed by this promise is not easy since it is hard to make the changes in one's life so he can be a blessing to the Lord God. If one walks down this path of wanting to bless the Lord God, there are innumerable blessings for him in terms of developing a growing closeness and intimacy with God. However, one comes under a barrage of demonic assault which makes this path somewhat difficult, and at times agonizing, until he learns from God how to deal with it; although our God is well able to deal with these attacks on our behalf.

How we can bless God

Blessing God is in many ways similar to blessing another person. At the end of this chapter one should have a broad understanding of what one must do to be a blessing to God. In turn He has spelled out the benefits He will give to those who do succeed in blessing Him (Psalm 103:1-5). Verse 2b states, "Forget not all His benefits." The Hebrew word for *forget* is related to a word which means "crippled." Thus, forgetting God's benefits cripples one.

Three things must be kept in mind when planning how we can bless God. These are that we cannot bless God with our ideas for

His mind is so far above ours in intellectual capacity that we in no way even approach it. The second is that He is our Father in the spiritual realm after we go through the second birth and thus we should look to Him for guidance. The third is that He owns the creation and all of the wealth in it so there is nothing that we can offer to Him in material substance. God does have men offer Him their substance, but this is really for the benefit of the one offering so that he can learn the blessings in giving to others. God uses this to train His children and not to gain materially from it.

There are many things which God requires of His children, and the execution of these probably does not qualify in His mind as a blessing but rather as the fulfillment of a duty (Luke 17:6-10). It is when a person goes above and beyond the ordinary course of events that he is likely to bless the heart of our Heavenly Father. Below are some of the things that God requires of us, but that is not quite the same as blessing Him. We can never be certain whether particular actions of an individual will bless the Lord, but examination of the Scriptures will help us to understand how we can definitely bless the heart of God.

Summary of Scriptures pertaining to blessing God

The Scriptures are helpful, especially the Psalms, in showing how we can bless God. It is good to review the Scriptures on how we can bless God. We are going to look at these closely so that we can get a better idea of how we can bless God and obtain His benefits listed in Psalm 103:1-5. After this we will look at how we can change from the present state of our relationship with God to what is required to be a blessing to Him. This transition will take work and involves purifying our heart, renewing our minds, and cleansing our spirits. This does not happen overnight, but it is only as the Lord God looks down at one's heart that He will be blessed if it is a heart that fulfills these conditions. Deciding in our minds that we are going to bless God by talking with someone about Him may seem to us a good thing to do; but, changing to blessing Him with all of our soul (much more than our intellect) requires a profound change in our hearts; and few there are who seem willing to go through this change.

Matthew 10:39

[39] He that findeth his life shall lose it: and he that loseth his life for my sake shall find it.

A Study of Scripture shows the following to be a blessing to God:

1. Constantly call to remembrance the good things that the Lord has done for you individually and collectively.

2. Worship with bowed heads and give the sacrifice of praise in great and frequent amounts. The praise has to recount what God has done for you as an individual and as parts of groups in society. It frequently includes song. It can be loud. It has to be with the whole soul (body, heart, mind, and strength); so singing, dancing, and loudness will be frequently involved. Specifically we must salute Him by raising our hands.

3. Be glad for the Lord God.

4. Exalt God's character. This activity is above all else, including blessing and praise. Recall things He has done for you that demonstrate His character. A good list of His preferred behaviors can be found in the list of the fruit of the Spirit in Galatians 5. Let Him form the fruit of the Spirit in you.

5. We must be exalting Him all of the time by ALL of our actions, words, and thoughts. We must take all of these actions, words, and thoughts captive for the Lord Jesus Christ (2 Corinthians 10:5). This will be a blessing to Him.

6. Keep a list of all of the wonderful things with which God has blessed you, and keep them at the front of your memory, and be ready to tell others about them. Bless God by

telling Him how much these acts have blessed you.

7. Adore the Lord and His character (we will study His character later—power, emotions, and intellect).

8. All of the above can only flow out of a close association and relationship with God. One must know God well to even have a hope of blessing Him. Look at how willing He is to be blessed by the return home of the prodigal son. He came running to meet the son afar off. That is who God is.

9. Thank God by recounting the advice He has given you about many situations. Especially bless Him for His instructions in the night.

10. Set God before you at all times, and keep Him on your right side always. Turn to Him first with all situations and concerns.

11. Bless the Lord with all of the above in meeting as groups, such as in a church service, and in secular situations as He leads you to share with someone.

12. Praise God continually in all that you do, say, and think. Speak out these praises of what he has given you and done for you before others. The only boast one should make is in the glory of the Lord and the fact that he loves you. Magnify God before others all of the time. By these actions we show His salvation daily.

13. Psalm 100:4 is so important that we list it here: ⁴ Enter into his gates with thanksgiving, *and* into his courts with praise: be thankful unto him, *and* bless his name (synonym for character).

14. Be thankful unto Him in your heart and not just with your intellect. This requires purifying our heart and renewing our mind. We will discuss how to purify the heart and re-

new the mind later.

15. Psalm 103:1: [1] Bless the LORD, O my soul: and all that is within me, *bless* his holy name.

16. Bless the Lord God with all your strength, power, and might. You have to be contagiously enthusiastic. The rest of Psalm 103 and parts of 104 ask you to recall His benefits which flow from His character. This blesses the heart of God, as you recount how He has blessed you.

17. Bless the Lord always from now and forever, including praising Him continually for what he has done for you. You can do this by your actions, your thoughts, and your speech; BUT a lot of it involves the second-by-second state in which you keep our inner man (your spirit). You must worship God in your spirit and in truth; the Scriptures command this. You can only do this as we purify our heart and renew our mind. We will discuss how to do this later in some detail. You have to be consumed with your love for Him in your spirit and flesh. It is only as you mature in your spirit that you will know when your spirit is active instead of when your flesh is active. Before maturation of your spirit it is difficult to know when your spirit is active in your thoughts and actions.

18. Have your devotion to Him in obedience and worship such that your heart has the Lord Jesus Christ formed in it. Perhaps the greatest compliment you can pay to God is to want to be like Him (1 John 3:2). You should want to be like Him in every way and do all of the things that He did.

Galatians 4:19

[19] My little children, of whom I travail in birth again until Christ be formed in you.

Scripture references for the above list of eighteen points

Deuteronomy Chapter 8:10, 1 Chronicles 29:20–22, Psalm 16:7–9, Psalm 26:12, Psalm 34:1–3, Psalm 63:4, Psalm 66:8, Psalm 96:2, Psalm 115:18, Psalm 145:2, and Psalm 145:21

Scripture that suggests actions that are not at the level of a blessing to God but nonetheless are probably pleasing to Him

Luke 17:5–10

[5] And the apostles said unto the Lord, Increase our faith. [6] And the Lord said, If ye had faith as a grain of mustard seed, ye might say unto this sycamine tree, Be thou plucked up by the root, and be thou planted in the sea; and it should obey you. [7] But which of you, having a servant plowing or feeding cattle, will say unto him by and by, when he is come from the field, Go and sit down to meat? [8] And will not rather say unto him, Make ready wherewith I may sup, and gird thyself, and serve me, till I have eaten and drunken; and afterward thou shalt eat and drink? [9] Doth he thank that servant because he did the things that were commanded him? I trow not. [10] So likewise ye, when ye shall have done all those things which are commanded you, say, We are unprofitable servants: we have done that which was our duty to do.

Note that, if the servant does just that which is expected, this is not providing a blessing; and it is not increasing faith (which develops from a close relationship with God). Look at another Scripture in the Gospel of John.

John 14:15

[15] If ye love me, keep my commandments.

Contrast this to the First Commandment. If we break a commandment then we are showing that we do not love God as we should. The Ten Commandments are summed up in the first two commandments. They are much more foundational than a lot of other laws and practices that the Lord commanded, and this is something to which we must pay attention if we are to bless the heart of God.

To bless God, we must have been in a maturing relationship at a highly personal level over a period of time.

This is evident from the list above on what God counts as blessing Him.

People cited in Scripture who have blessed God

Moses became a friend of God and was described as the meekest man ever; but God still punished him for what, to many, would seem a minor infringement on one occasion when his temper broke forth.

Abraham was a friend of God. Enoch walked with God and did not see death. Elijah also walked with God and did not see death. King David had one thing which God held against him, the matter of Uriah, the Hittite; otherwise God described him as a man after His own heart.

How to bless God

When we bless God according to the manner presented above and do so in our spirit and heart (we will cover more soon about the differences among the mind, the spirit, and the heart) then we will find that we start to get the blessings in Psalm 103:1-5. God keeps His Word and will meet us over halfway as we see in the account of the prodigal son. Although God would like perfection in us He does not expect it. He does, however, expect a consuming effort on our part.

The Church in the West

The present state of many of the nations in the West is similar. There is a decreasing interest in God; the churches have become very weak in spiritual power and strength, having gravitated toward a situation seen in the chirch of Laodicea described in Revelation. The church is neither hot nor cold and is not blessing God. It is in danger of being trodden down as salt which has lost its savor. The church is, in a sense, the sum of its members. It is far from the description of God's expectations for it.

God's wishes and vision for the Church, as described in the Scriptures:

a. Having power for delivering miracles at individual levels

b. Having power to survive persecution and to thrive

c. Being a body closely knit with its head, the Lord Jesus Christ

d. Working with the head in order to take back the works of the devil

e. Performing a ministry of reconciling to God those who will be reconciled

f. Preaching and teaching, not be from mental prowess of the preacher or teacher in intellectual understanding, but rather through demonstration of spiritual power, revelation, knowledge, prophesy, and true doctrine (not worldly wisdom), all of which can come only from a dynamic relationship with its head, the Lord Jesus Christ

g. Having all members in a dynamic relationship with the Lord Jesus Christ, the head of the body

God has given various spiritual gifts to the individual members; and He has given apostles, prophets, evangelists, and pastor/teachers as a gift to the body. All of the work of the Church is subject to its being worked through the love of God, which is not just an emotion but rather is a great and powerful spirit with intent and purpose, enormous emotional intensity, and great power in the spiritual realm.

How to change from the present state of the Church to that which will bless God

We will answer this issue of change in the next several chapters. For now, we note that there is great change needed in the Church organization and function; the hearts and spirits of many in Church leadership; and the training of the members. The clearly-stated goal in the Scripture below is not being achieved by the present structure, organization, and training. God expects the stature and fullness of Christ is His standard.

Ephesians 4:11–13

[11] And he gave some, apostles; and some, prophets; and some, evangelists; and some, pastors and teachers; [12] For the perfecting of the saints, for the work of the ministry, for the edifying of the body of Christ: [13] Till we all come in the unity of the faith, and of the knowledge of the Son of God, unto a perfect man, unto the measure of the stature of the fulness of Christ.

There are several regarding this change:

1. One question is how does an individual progress and change from an intellect-driven faith, which is neither hot nor cold, to the powerful and emotionally-driven purposeful life in our God as a thriving branch in a powerful vine? As individuals change, they become the building blocks of a rehabilitated body; and we believe that our God wants this. As this transition comes about, there will be much more healing both spiritually and physically. At the same time as individuals change, there must be a change at the leadership level of the churches to let God speak His plan into the hearts of individual members. The Church leadership has to correct many wrong decisions and understandings that have come into the Church over the last three hundred years. We will discuss these wrong decisions in brief in Chapter 8. In this book we are trying to help people at the individual level to receive spiritual and physical

healing from our Lord God. The Church, corporately, also needs spiritual and physical healing. Therefore we have to have change both in individuals and in the structure and organization of the Church in order to bless God.

2. Spiritual and physical disease and healing are knit in an unbreakable bond. One cannot have one without the other. This is because of the need for spiritual power to bring healing. We are used to looking at great displays of power in our natural world—such as great aircraft, powerful explosive devices including nuclear weapons, and gigantic machinery. If all of these are multiplied millions of times, they are infinitesimally small compared with the spiritual power God used in forming this creation and that He uses in maintaining it (Hebrews 1:3 and 11:3). We will review these in more detail later. We must have the power of God working in the Church and in individuals in order to bless God.

3. In order to make this huge transition from one's current state to that of having spiritual power and being under the Lord God's guidance and direction moment by moment, we have to look at what God states in His Word and then allow Him to work with us as individuals in a vital relationship with Him. We will have to understand the structure and function of the spiritual man to co-opetate with God in changing individuals and the Church. The details of the spiritual man are prominent in Scripture but have been missed by many for a long time. They have been fully discussed in our previous book, *How to be Led by the Spirit of God*. In a sense we have to learn to communicate with God. Many people think that by praying to God they are communicating with Him. This is only a small part of what He wants. In both the Old and the New Covenants God requires each individual to be able to hear His voice and interpret His actions.

We are going to review the building blocks in the next chapters which allow God to bring about His purposes and changes in each individual. It is only as one allows God to change him that he will ever feel a true sense of purpose and fulfillment. This is because God has put a desire for these things deeply within each of us; and they are still there but suppressed below the level of awareness by busy lives, suffering and emotional trauma, and many false doctrines and knowledge in our societies. As individuals heal, the Church will start to heal. Therefore, we need to look at the steps involved for individuals' healing. The healing that God longs to give to all is for each to reach his destiny in Him.

We have noted that God told Bruce in 1998 that the churches were weak. One might need to seek good teaching through alternative outlets until the current church leadership starts to address mounting deficiencies in the approach it has used to feeding God's flock. In selecting any teaching ministry which supports the Church, one needs to have discernment about the message being imparted (is it truth?). Also he should ideally know that God is blessing it.

Steps to take in order to come into a dynamic relationship with God

The steps are all integrated together with each individual's forming a dynamic relationship with God. We are going to state the steps in numerical points here, and then we will discuss them in the following chapters.

At that point one should have a roadmap for how to work with God, through His methods, to undergo the personal change that is needed. As one changes, he will be healed spiritually of many breaches in his spirit; and physical healing will occur as the power of God's Spirit flows through that person into the surrounding community as love being shed abroad through the heart.

Romans 5:5

[5] And hope maketh not ashamed; because the love of God is shed

abroad in our hearts by the Holy Ghost which is given unto us.

We will cover the following points, listed in abbreviated form, in the following chapters:

1. We need to understand God's character (power, motivations, emotions, and intellect); and we need to understand why He made the creation to include illness and death. If one is looking to God for healing, then he will want to gain confidence in God's willingness to heal, and God's ability to heal.

2. We need to understand God's purpose for illness in the creation and also how He uses it for His purposes in the creation.

3. We need to understand the power in the Spirit of God in order to understand the structure of the creation and why all natural wisdom is false. Grasping this will help one to begin living in the spiritual realm, which is what God wants for those who have been through the second birth.

4. We have to understand the differences between hope, faith, and belief. We also need to understand when belief is in the heart and not just in the mind. We have to understand how to develop belief in the heart from an idea in the mind.

5. We have to understand that God wants His people to work with Him, as co-laborers in this age and in the future ages, and how He prepares them for this role.

6. We have to understand the full meaning of the second birth (born again). This involves learning how to live in the spiritual realm and not just to live in the natural realm.

7. We need to understand true wisdom, understanding, and knowledge as opposed to false wisdom, understanding, and knowledge—relating to the relationship and interac-

tions of the spiritual and natural realms. This is important for understanding the relationship between the spirit and the flesh in each individual. It is reflected in the health of the flesh and spirit.

8. We need to understand the structure of spiritual man since it preceded and led to the structure of natural man. It is critical to study this since it allows one to understand how to work with God to make needed changes for spiritual and natural healing.

9. We have to understand the pathways to maturing in the spiritual inner man. The flesh needs to be subdued in all of its evil intent; and several things need to occur—purification of the heart, cleansing of the spirit, renewal of the mind, elimination of self will, and how to praise, worship, and bless God in the spirit and in truth. These acts are opposed to those acts being done in flesh and in "false truth."

10. We need to understand when God, the Father and the Lord Jesus Christ become resident in the human heart. Their presence brings the full presence of God to the individual.

When one understands these things, he will have an intellectual understanding of the steps involved in the changing. Then he will be in a very good position to start working with God toward spiritual maturity. This will result in power over the flesh with all of the healing energy and will of God directed toward healing him and those in his sphere of influence. The healing must first be in the spirit; then, if the appropriate changes are made, it will begin to manifest in the flesh.

These are the points that we will develop in the next several chapters. It will only be as one applies the concepts personally that he will mature in his spirit, will bless God, and will be healed of all of his diseases.

God's Character revealed in attitudes and emotions and The Spiritual Heart

Chapter 3

Introduction

At the end of the last chapter we listed a number of topics which we need to discuss in order to give the reader a framework which will enable him to work with God in order to make internal changes in his mind, heart, and spirit such that he can mature in his spirit and eventually be a blessing to God. The greatest need for all of God's children (adopted through the second birth) is to understand His character through interaction with Him throughout many personal experiences. This is entirely different from repeating set of phrases such as "God is love"; "God is good." Both are true but do not help the person using them to know God truly. There are great blessings listed in Scripture for those who come to know God's character through working with Him over time. Those in Psalm 91:14-16 are very strong. Remember that in Hebrew a persons name indicates his character.

Psalm 91:14–16

[14] Because he hath set his love upon me, therefore will I deliver him: I will set him on high, because he hath known my name. [15] He shall call upon me, and I will answer him: I *will be* with him in trouble; I will deliver him, and honour him. [16] With long life will I satisfy him, and shew him my salvation.

Knowing the character of God builds up trust and also is a strong defense to the vicious attacks against truth that evil spirits bring to us. In order to start us thinking more about the wonderful and loving; all powerful; and intellectually incredible God that we have for our heavenly Father let us review what he is like through His actions and statements.

God's Character

When we turn to a physician for healing, we are just being wise if we seek references from those who have been treated by him in order to find out about his capabilities and character. When one contemplates turning to God for healing the same questions should arise. We understand God's capabilities and character as we get to know Him better.

Many people look to God for healing as a "long-shot" that would be wonderful if it works out. They may not express it like that; but many who seek God for healing really know very little about Him and have had few interactions with Him that allow a close knowledge. Bruce, driving home from work one evening in 2007, was musing about why we see so few healings by God in the U.S.A. As Bruce mused, the Holy Spirit said: "People want faith for healing, but they do not want faith in me." That is so like many whom the Lord Jesus Christ healed during His advent. Nine of ten with leprosy never returned to express thanks (Luke 17:12).

When we are discussing healing by God, we are not talking about the confusing situation of one seeking medical assistance and then attributing the healing to God. We discussed earlier that these are different. We should be grateful to God for providing medical knowledge in our society for pain relief and many other health conditions. In this chapter we are going to introduce the reader to a God about whom he probably spends very little time thinking, an issue which will be to his eternal loss.

God's works are seen best when one is living primarily in the spiritual realm.

When one wants to study God's character and His power, it is helpful to consider His works since these reveal much about Him. Recall that God is spirit, and without the second birth and subsequent maturation all we can see of Him are the effects of His works in this natural realm. God cursed the whole creation when Adam and Eve broke fellowship in the Garden of Eden and He

withdrew His life-giving spirit from the creation. He also condemned men to eternal separation from His life-giving spirit. This
is spiritual death (the second death). The things we see and observe with our natural senses are confined to the created realm.
This realm is without life, except for those places and people God
has touched in His ministry of reconciliation. This ministry of
reconciliation of people to Him is His, and He uses it to restore
fellowship with those who will respond to Him and seek Him.
At the point God chooses to restore fellowship (only He can do
this—John 1:13) He gives that individual a new spiritual heart
and a new spirit. He writes His laws in the heart and mind, and
the Holy Spirit indwells the new spiritual heart. The new spirit is
of God and from God.

This event is the second birth and is well discussed in the Gospel
of John, chapter 3. Many people think that the second birth is an
emotional experience one goes through after which he is granted
eternal life and will live in heaven with God for eternity. The second birth is much more than this. Since this is little understood,
few seek to differently after the second birth and return to their
former state of a flesh-dominated life. They have little spiritual
development and confine their worship to the flesh and mind, instead of worshiping in spirit and in truth.

The second birth is so much greater than this. It is a birth of a new
inner man into a new realm with different laws of operation and
where time is not the same so that the so-called observed natural
laws of space and time have no predictive ability. This inner man
has a similar set of senses to the natural man and only God, as our
spiritual Father, is able to teach us how to use them and to show
us what we are seeing and hearing. We can mature in the spiritual
realm only as we work very closely with God. Spiritual-realm
knowledge is not derived analytically, and there is little or no application of natural realm-knowledge in the spiritual realm. We
soon come to realize that anything not revealed by God through
prophecy, knowledge, revelation, His written Word the Bible as
taught by the Holy Spirit, or by His power is false. The enor-

mity of the falseness of ideas and concepts in the natural realm is hard to grasp, and many will resist this statement. However, when one considers all of the miracles that defied the natural laws of physics, chemistry, and mechanics, he will realize that these laws all break down in the presence of a spiritual-realm act. So-called natural laws operate much of the time but all should be presented with the disclaimer that they will not be accurate in the presence of spiritual-realm power unleashed by God or powerful angels.

The new man after the second birth is called to renew his mind so that the complete focus is on using spiritual senses to live in the spiritual realm with God. That involves listening and seeing with the inner man and depending on the truth of this over what one sees and hears with the natural senses. It is only as one lives in this spiritual realm (that is, makes it and the laws which govern it primary foci of all his decisions) that he can see God's character and His power much more clearly.

God gave Bruce a botanical analogy. Since God cursed it, the natural realm is like a flower that is dehydrated, wilted, and at the end of its existence. When the Spirit of God touches it and brings life to it as He flows through it, the flower becomes totally different. It becomes alive in a way that one could never have foreseen using just natural realm-knowledge.

We in our natural bodies of flesh are like the wilted flower with the strong odor of death, the abnormal chemistry, and the hugely-distorted structure. The whole natural-realm part of the creation is like this also. Our natural laws of physics and material science are applicable only to this dead and dying natural realm. When one goes through the second birth but does not mature, then there will be little flow of God's Spirit through him; and he will remain very much like the wilted flower, although there would be a flicker of life. God's expectation is that the redeemed man will start a deep and intense relationship with Him and that the flow of the Spirit of God into him will be an exhibit like a lighthouse and he will emit the light of God into a natural realm, which is almost completely devoid of the light of God. It is the duty of the Church to prepare new spiritual infants to relate to God but sadly this is rarely done. As a result, in Western societies there is little evidence for the incredibly intense life—emotion, intellect, and power—seen in the people of God. The church tries to substitute intellectual development for spiritual power and maturation and the two are not akin.

God's purposes for making the creation the way He did

God made the history of the creation such that it would fulfill His desires for it. He knew what the outcome of alternative histories would be in great detail, as can be seen in the Scripture below. It shows that God knew what alternative histories would be like even for a small town which at a specific time in history.

Matthew 11:21

[21] Woe unto thee, Chorazin! woe unto thee, Bethsaida! for if the mighty works, which were done in you, had been done in Tyre and Sidon, they would have repented long ago in sackcloth and ashes.

Purposes for God's redeemed People

There are purposes for God's redeemed people (those given the second birth) both in this period of history and in the eternal ages to come. Some of these are:

a. To reveal God to the rest of mankind—showing His character, His plans, and His power (requiring them to be in the correct relationship with God in order to represent Him in truth)

b. To provide a bride for His son

c. To be a special family to rule and to reign with God in the ages to come

d. To fulfill the general obligations for all mankind

God purposed to create in such a way that it would please Him.

Revelation 4:11

[11] Thou art worthy, O Lord, to receive glory and honour and power: for thou hast created all things, and for thy pleasure they are and were created.

God is more than willing to give pleasure to those He created if they will accept His good intentions for them. The creation serves in a way as a training area for God's redeemed people to prepare them for the ages to come. This is shown by the scripture about the vessels (people). Our choices in this phase of life set our future in the eternal ages.

2 Timothy 2:20

[20] But in a great house there are not only vessels of gold and of silver, but also of wood and of earth; and some to honour, and some to dishonour.

What scriptures reveal about God's character

God chose to sacrifice His Son, the Lord Jesus Christ, to redeem willing individuals from a life in eternity separated from Him. This was an incredible sacrifice, and God will set his face like flint against those who spurn it. However, He will not be pleased by their going into death apart from Him. In the sacrifice on the cross of the Lord Jesus Christ, God demonstrated how much He loved the people of the world. No other act could have been this hard for a God who has an intense love for His Son. If we were in similar circumstances, we could still little imagine the emotional suffering of God and of His Son, because our emotional strength is quite weak in comparison with that of God. The Lord Jesus Christ in allowing His father to reconcile fallen mankind through His advent and death, forever emptied Himself from the complete power and resources that He had before. He is God and man at the same time but He is now limited to having the body of a man for eternity (Philippians 2:5-11).

God is not pleased by the death of any unredeemed man, and He constantly strives to win each soul until a point that He can see that the individual will not allow that. God comes running to meet the prodigal children from afar off as soon as each one sets his face to return to God.

God's spirit expresses the positive unifying emotions preferentially. He acts in judgment and in burning with an eternal (non-consuming purifying) fire only after all recourse has been declined by an individual. He respects each person's choice for his eternal habitation. There will be dwellings in the Lake of Fire, and individuals will be able to socialize; but the environment will be one of torment.

Truth is a foundation of God's character (Psalm 146:6). Truth sets the foundation and framework for the creation. When the demonic spirits try to build on the negative separating emotions, they use lies and fear. There is no substance or strength in these structures, and they cannot stand against truth.

God is a servant to His people.

God will supply all needs for His people now and in eternity

God will dwell with His people in eternity.

The seven spirits of God express His character attributes. We briefly discuss these in our book *Spirit*. God describes His character in His YWHW compound names in a progressive revelation from Genesis to Revelation (See Alta Ada's new book *The Character of God as revealed in His YHWH Compound Names*).

God is unchanging and does not favor one person over another in terms of the chance he has to succeed. If one has more talents given then more is expected of him.

God's judgments are just.

God's love when experienced is a force so powerful that it would crush and fold a person into one with God if it were not attenuated by God. The joy of God and His kindness are palpable.

He is kind, and long suffering (evidenced by the centuries He spent trying to appeal to Israel to return to Him prior to the Babylonian exile).

God is merciful.

God can envelope a person in a spirit of joy and peace that is palpable when present.

Distortion of God's Character

The devil and his demons have built a fabric of lies and distortions in this natural realm over which they currently rule. They do not rule over those who have been through the second birth but they do all that they can to neutralize the impact of these people.

There is a demonic hierarchy of powers which integrates with men in a structure to support the objectives of these demons who serve under Satan and his agenda. The agenda is essentially to defy God within the rules in which He has allowed them to operate.

These demons have released throughout history various philosophies and have controlled education systems. They have posed as many false deities through history (cp Psalm 106:37 and Psalm 106:38). They rely on God's overall ruling of the entire creation in such a way that no man is coerced by Him into making any choice which is not freely made. Using this they constantly bring accurate accusations before God using material against God's adopted children.

Revelation 12:10

[10] And I heard a loud voice saying in heaven, Now is come salvation, and strength, and the kingdom of our God, and the power of his Christ: for the accuser of our brethren is cast down, which accused them before our God day and night.

These evil spirits inflict coercing spiritual, emotional, and intellectual forces on men to attempt to thwart God's plans to redeem men, and to neutralize any work they may do for God after they have been redeemed.

God's character has been so distorted in current Western society that one is reminded of the marring of the Lord Jesus Christ physically to where He was not recognizable (leading up to the crucifixion – [Isaiah 52:14]).

God's Word

God's Word is His revealed truth, and it sets both the physical and the moral operating boundaries of the creation for eternity. In the Bible God has answered every single questions that all of His people will ever have in this age because He foresaw all of their questions before the foundation of the world. It was before the foundation of the world that the sacrifice of the Lord Jesus Christ took place in the spiritual realm, and eventually it was performed in the natural realm (hence the need to pray for God's will to be done on earth as it is in heaven). The timing in the two realms is not the same. The whole concept of time in the spiritual realm is different from that in the natural realm. One has to search the Scriptures for specific answers to many questions. Of course answers to such issues as to what color car to buy are answered in the sense that the rules are provided for getting answers from God to such specific concerns. There is much in the Scriptures related to how to live and function in both the natural and spiritual realms.

God's emotions

God has the same range of emotions as people, since man was made in His image. The emotions of God are without guile. They are pure and are used to address specific situations. They are never manipulative or coercive. In comparison with those of an individual they are enormously powerful and can move the whole creation. King David in Psalm 18 describes the anger of God and the impact of His anger on the earth. God's anger led Him to perform further acts described in verses 8-13.

Psalm 18:6–7

In my distress I called upon the LORD, and cried unto my God: he heard my voice out of his temple, and my cry came before him, *even* into his ears. [7] Then the earth shook and trembled; the foundations also of the hills moved and were shaken, because he was wroth.

The power in God's love is evidenced by the following Scripture.

Romans 8:38-39

For I am persuaded, that neither death, nor life, nor angels, nor principalities, nor powers, nor things present, nor things to come, [39] Nor height, nor depth, nor any other creature, shall be able to separate us from the love of God, which is in Christ Jesus our Lord.

Essentially, nothing can separate God's people from His love. We must remember that, even when we close off our receptors from experiencing this love, it is still there. No demonic force can separate us from God's powerful love. No structures we erect within our own spiritual hearts can separate us from His love. The whole passage in Romans chapter 8: 28-39 speaks of the power of the emotional force in God's love. It is a force stronger than any physical force between atoms and molecules in the nuclear weapons on earth, and we say that in an advised and absolutely literal manner, for it is true.

The following scripture shows that no demon can stand against the power of the emotional force known as God's love. If we allow our spiritual heart to be purified under God's supervision, then there will be such a force inside it that it will squeeze out the influence of even the most powerful of demons. We are not talking about demonic possession of the heart. Demons can influence hearts from afar in large geographic areas (Daniel 10:13). We will discuss further in Chapter 7 how demons exert spiritual power to influence men.

1 John 4:18

There is no fear in love; but perfect love casteth out fear: because fear hath torment. He that feareth is not made perfect in love.

To have the love of God perfected in the heart is one of the best ways of being healed of all disease caused by demons.

God's Character, His use of illness, and His willingness to perform spiritual and physical Healing

God states early in the Bible that He is the God Who heals. This is where He first uses His name YHWH Rapha. This indicates the desire to heal is a deep and eternal character attribute. We have to block Him from healing by our lack of faith, lack of belief, or our behavior. If faith, belief, and behavior meet His demands then God will heal. The Scripture Exodus 15:26 (below) also indicates that frequently we have illnesses given by God in order to make us realize that we are not in the relationship with Him that we should be. It is a warning to save us from eternal separation from Him; or if we have been through the second birth, He may challenge us to improve our relationship with Him. Allowing God to fill our hearts with love would not cause the healing of such illnesses; but by the time He did this He would have healed us of diseases that He placed on us, since to be filled with God's love our hearts have to be purified.

Exodus 15:26

[26] And said, If thou wilt diligently hearken to the voice of the LORD thy God, and wilt do that which is right in his sight, and wilt give ear to his commandments, and keep all his statutes, I will put none of these diseases upon thee, which I have brought upon the Egyptians: for I *am* the LORD that healeth thee.

God commanded the Israelites to learn individually to hear Him speaking to them. If one cannot hear or see an individual, then there is very little in the relationship. The same applies to people who have not learned how to listen to and to observe God acting in their lives. The Lord Jesus Christ repeated the need for individuals to be obedient to God; to do this they must hear and see His communications to them.

If we do not obey God's instructions (voice), then we follow demonic spirits; or we follow our impulses of our flesh, which God has judged as evil and worthy of eternal death. There are only a limited number of places that our thoughts originate. We deal with this extensively in our book *How to be Led by the Spirit of God: Maturing in the Spirit*. Later, we will look at a brief summary of the structure of our soul, and then we will learn more about the spirit and the flesh. We will also look more closely at how God speaks to us and how we can learn to communicate with Him. Proverbs 4:20-22 show the benefits received by reading Scripture and by listening to and seeing God's communications with us.

Proverbs 4:20–22

My son, attend to my words; incline thine ear unto my sayings. Let them not depart from thine eyes; keep them in the midst of thine heart. For they *are* life unto those that find them, and health [*lit.*, medicine] to all their flesh.

This Scripture is very important and tells us to study diligently the Scriptures under the teachings of the Holy Spirit, to listen to God, and to talk with God. God says to keep His Word constantly before us. When we do this, all of our flesh will be healthy; and we will have eternal life. This is another magnificent promise to God's people.

Further consideration of the relation between sin and sickness

Matthew 9:6

⁶ But that ye may know that the Son of man hath power on earth to forgive sins, (then saith he to the sick of the palsy,) Arise, take up thy bed, and go unto thine house.

Psalms 38 and 39 show the impact of sin on illness in King David's experience. 1 Timothy 1:20 to see how God will use the demonic forces to teach people to avoid sin patterns.

The Lord Jesus Christ constantly equated sickness with sin. We have to repent if we want to be healed. This does not mean God will not heal us without that step, but it makes it uncertain as to whether He will.

So much does God desire for His children to have healing in their flesh of sickness and infirmity that He actually commands it (Hebrews 12:5-13, esp v. 13). If we disobey God, we do not lose salvation; but we will be saved through fire (1 Corinthians 3:13-15). Let us look more closely at this situation. We believe God commands healing of a person in order for Him to allow him to get into a close proximity to God. This is shown in the case of the woman who touched the hem of the Lord Jesus' garment. There is a strong relationship between God's wanting someone in close proximity to Him and His need to heal them. This is shown partly in Hebrews 12:5-13.

The healing power of God

Matthew 9:20

²⁰ And, behold, a woman, which was diseased with an issue of blood twelve years, came behind *him*, and touched the hem of his

garment.

This woman had watched the Lord healing other people, and she had come to a firm conviction that His power to heal would come to her body through touch. The Lord Jesus was aware that power flowed out of Him; BUT HE did not specifically plan this release of His power. This shows the healing nature of the power in God's Spirit, for healing results just from the flow of His Spirit into the person. If we come into His presence through praise and worship frequently and continually, we will have that same healing power flowing through us to the extent that our hearts are purified. Impure hearts block the flow of His Spirit to our flesh. One can read much more detail about this in our first book *How to be Led by the Spirit of God*.

Proximity and relationship to God bring His healing power into a person, and in His presence no illness or infirmity can continue. His power is so much more focused and delicate than anything men can replicate; it reaches from the microscopic molecular level all the way up to the astronomical level. And yet His power is enough to have formed the creation. At the end of History He will roll the creation up as a vesture (garment—see Hebrews 1:10-12), and make a new heaven and a new earth. His power is full of life, for He is a life-giving spirit. In this dying creation men rarely see the life-giving power of God in action; to see it is life-changing.

His character and power are such that all who believe can pull that power from Him into their situation. One does not even need to be in physical proximity to God, as other healing miracles demonstrate that he can order those under Him (angels) to deliver healing. In addition, men to whom He has delegated His power, for the purpose of healing are able to bring the Lord's healing to other people.

When the Lord commands healing in Hebrews 12:13, He is in a sense commanding closeness of relationship to Him. The Scriptures tell us that if we make the first move in drawing close to God, He will come running to meet us ("draw nigh unto God and

He will draw nigh unto you").

God has described many ways His children (people who are re-deemed and have received the second birth) can receive healing. All depend on being obedient to His individual utterances to them and to His written words in the Bible. The passage on healing in James 5:13-16 states that the prayer of faith will save the sick. Faith comes only from God's individual utterances to individuals. Frequently faith comes from a Scripture passage that the Holy Spirit emphasizes.

Romans 10:17

[17] So then faith *cometh* by hearing, and hearing by the word of God.

There is no other way that faith comes, and without faith it is impossible to please God (Hebrews 11:6). There are two words in Greek for the English word *word*. One is *logos* for the writ-ten Scripture and for the incarnate Word, Jesus; and the other is *rhema* for the individual spoken communications. The hearing mentioned in this Scripture (Romans 10:17) is of the individual utterance of God to an individual.

Therefore, if one wants to be assured of healing, one has to pursue an individual relationship with God where he is able to bless God by following His individual instructions to him as He purifies his heart. When this occurs, we are assured that God will heal. We must be careful to judge our own hearts correctly in order to claim this Scripture below.

Psalm 103:1–3

[1] Bless the LORD, O my soul: and all that is within me, *bless* his holy name. [2] Bless the LORD, O my soul, and forget not all his benefits: [3] Who forgiveth all thine iniquities; who healeth all thy diseases.

God will heal us if our soul blesses Him. That is a sure promise.

We looked at what blesses God in Chapter Two. Proverbs 4:20-22 is also a sure promise for how to be blessed by God with physical healing.

The Spiritual Heart

We have mentioned the spiritual heart frequently and will now elaborate on what it is, since the way that God sees an individual is largely based on the content and nature of his spiritual heart. Therefore, our spiritual heart will play a large role in whether we can receive healing from God and whether He will release His power to us for healing the flesh and the spirit. Proverbs 27:19 shows us that God sees the spiritual heart (our core) as who we are before Him. Therefore, it is very important to understand it thoroughly. We will provide a summary here; but for more discussion one can read our book *How to be Led by the Spirit of God: Maturing in the Spirit.*

Proverbs 27:19

[19] As in water face *answereth* to face, so the heart of man to man.

Description of the spiritual heart

The heart cannot be described in natural realm understanding, since, unlike the heart of the flesh, it does not occupy a specific anatomical location in the flesh. We have diagrammed it in our book *Spirit*. That diagram is based on Scripture which shows that our inner man fits into the flesh like a sword into a sheath (Daniel 7:15). Since our inner man lives in the spiritual heart (1 Peter 3:4), then we understand that the heart also occupies a position following the contours of the body of flesh and is surrounding the spirit.

God made the spiritual heart to convey His Spirit to our flesh and to the community around us. The life is in the blood (Leviticus 17:14); therefore, the spirit circulates in the blood and is in the spiritual heart. These two statements are consistent. The natural heart nourishes the cells of the body by circulating blood with nutrients to them in order to maintain a state gradually dying from birth. The spiritual heart circulates the spiritual nutrients which are vitally essential for our soul and inner man to grow in strength and to mature. The spiritual heart also allows for the love of God to be shed abroad (Romans 5:5) when the Holy Spirit begins to reside in the heart after the second birth.

Within our heart reside a lot of spiritual buildings and pathways which contain our beliefs and attitudes and which organize our behavioral responses to all incoming information. We are responsible to God for what we build and maintain in our hearts. Before the second birth everything we built was to serve the flesh. God literally had to break through a lot of barricades to make us look at good and evil as a means to start us looking to Him, prior to His giving us the second birth.

At the time of the second birth we were given a new heart, but it shortly falls into the ways of the old heart due to our failure to renew our minds. The degree to which it falls back varies between individuals. For most of us, unless we have undertaken a deliberate purification of our heart under the direction of the Holy Spirit, our heart will almost certainly contain many impurities and a lot of false wisdom, understanding, and knowledge. We will have many unholy attitudes, beliefs, and behaviors. Many of the devices we have erected are laid by the flesh as a barricade against the love of God permeating our flesh and the surrounding community.

Concepts which may help to understand the heart

Think of the heart as a city built on a particular landscape and in a particular geography. The heart of each person is unique in the combination. Our soul, using its mind, cannot see into the deepest parts of this city. This city has a mind of its own. This mind is operated upon by various parts of the flesh and at times (frequently) the influence of evil spirits using the flesh and its lusts to accomplish their own purposes (this has nothing to do with demonic possession). This mind of the heart is always subject to the mind of the soul in terms of expressing its thoughts but in much speaking the heart content is revealed. We can tell what is in our hearts by listening to our own words.

Matthew 12:34–37

[34] O generation of vipers, how can ye, being evil, speak good things? for out of the abundance of the heart the mouth speaketh. [35] A good man out of the good treasure of the heart bringeth forth good things: and an evil man out of the evil treasure bringeth forth evil things. [36] But I say unto you, That every idle word that men shall speak, they shall give account thereof in the day of judgment. [37] For by thy words thou shalt be justified, and by thy words thou shalt be condemned.

In this city within the heart our soul walks about. We stop here and there to admire an idol (all things raised up against God in the use of our time and our resources). We rest and contemplate good and bad past times. We sit and imagine a future. We form our deepest plans. We have beliefs about our lives, about our friends and family, about God, about our work, and about many other things. These are all stored in various buildings and along various paths. There are areas in each of our cities that we fear to tread. There are areas which may be quite dangerous and doors we hesitate to open.

In this city, as we give Him permission, God will build refuges, fortresses, and strong towers into which our soul can go (Psalm 61:3, Proverbs 18:10, and Psalm 91:1). These are buildings made in our hearts by the Word of God in which we can be protected when under attack from the enemy. They are spiritual buildings which prevent the weapons of the evil spirits from harming us.

Whenever any information comes into this city from the various roads into it (our physical senses and our spiritual senses when we have developed them), our city forms a response based on the past and which is organized by various members of this city (our many lusts and our many desires). Information is coming in all of the time. Usually we respond reflexively, based on past similar situations. Our heart sends a suggested behavior to the mind of the soul about what to say to and do about all incoming information. The mind of the soul has to sort out where this information originated—in the flesh, in the heart, or in the new spirit. Unless the mind of the soul is actively assessing all of these incoming thoughts from the heart, in order to renew itself, then it will just accept the content of the speech or the plan for behavior from the heart. The conscience will usually send a suggestion to the mind of the soul as the information moves from the heart to the mind of the soul. It is the mind of the soul which has to decide whether to allow the new spirit to express; or just to allow the flesh to express. Over time the flesh or the new spirit will strengthen and the other will weaken since a soul, through the mind of the soul, can decide whether to strengthen his inner man by deciding in his favor or to strengthen his flesh by default (Galatians 5:16-18).

The mind of the soul is better able to know what information is from the spirit as this mind of the soul is renewed (more about this later) and as the heart is purified. Both of these processes, the renewal of the mind and the purification of the heart need to be directed by God's speaking to each individual and directing the breaking down and removal of old structures, buildings, roads, and ruins. There will be a lot of decay, rust, and slime to remove. There will be nasty spirits unleashed in these processes of purifying the heart and renewing the mind. These two processes have to be coordinated by the Lord God; we are not clever enough, and we are not strong enough to outwit the demonic forces which will be unleashed when a person commits to God to do this.

Think carefully about doing this, and do it only as God directs when you give Him permission. He will bring situations and circumstances to you to make you see what needs to be changed; and you can agree at each decision point. If you do not allow God to build the house (structures in the city) and to guard the city, then whatever you do outside of God is empty as far as being of any eternal value or of any use in resisting the evil spirits when they arrack. We will discuss this further in Chapter 7.

Psalm 127:1

[1] Except the LORD build the house, they labour in vain that build it: except the LORD keep the city, the watchman waketh *but* in vain.

One should realize that without renewing the mind and purifying the heart a person is not likely to be a vessel of silver or gold in eternity. If a person commits to working with God, there will be no turning back (for God is not pleased by this). God is more than able to give one all victory over the demonic assault that will occur. He is so much more powerful than the devil, who can do nothing without God's permission. God uses the demonic spirits to train us for His eternal Kingdom (Job 1:6-12; and 1 Timothy 1:20). In these processes of change in our heart and mind, if we stay close to God (Psalm 91:1), then we have nothing to fear from these spirits; but we must be careful to listen to God, to do as He says, and to do what He shows us in order to change successfully.

The foundations in our heart

All of the structures of the flesh and unpurified heart are built on sand and are unstable when major external events occur. Both the man of the flesh and the man with a second birth without spiritual growth will have limited response to and limited ability to cope with many events. Their buildings will come tumbling down with the natural realm storms, floods, fires, and earthquakes in one's life. Absolutely nothing that we build in our heart in the natural realm, which uses the flesh and evil spirits, will stand. The spiritual-realm structures built on God's Word (without our own thoughtful but error-prone additions) will stand. The spiritual realm is far superior to the natural and is always in control of the natural realm within those guidelines which have been detailed in God's Word. We will look in more detail in Chapter 7 at the processes of tearing down old structures designed to prevent our receiving God and His Word into our hearts and the building of new structures founded on spiritual-realm truth and based soundly on God's Word alone (built on the Rock).

The buildings in our hearts

There is a very close relationship between words and spiritual structures. We are going to be accountable to God for every idle word we speak (Matthew 12:36); James 3:4-13 also addresses our spoken words. Our words and imaginations build and reveal the structures in our hearts. In many ways our words are our lives, and we live in our words. Scriptures such as Psalm 91:9 become much more meaningful for we make our habitation in the structures built by God's words when we trust them and believe them.

Psalm 91:9

[9] Because thou hast made the LORD, *which is* my refuge, *even* the most High, thy habitation;

God's words give structure throughout the ages to come and allow us to understand some of the issues which will be present in eternity. Throughout eternity the Lord's words will never pass away.

Matthew 24:35

[35] Heaven and earth shall pass away, but my words shall not pass away.

We must be very careful of all of our words at all times and to all people. Renewing the mind should make us more aware of the need to be careful with our speech.

Renewal of the mind and purification of the heart

As one submits to God to organize the destruction and the removal of the old attitudes, beliefs, behaviors, false wisdom, false understanding, and false knowledge, He will start to build on the

Rock (the Lord Jesus Christ), who is the truth. One will feel and hear in the spirit satisfying "clunks and thunks" as the Holy Spirit erects strong towers, fortresses, and refuges in the spiritual heart. Eventually, if the heart is purified sufficiently, the Father and the Son will come to dwell with him (John 14:23). At that point a person has the Holy Trinity abiding in him. How glorious this will be!

John 14:23

[23] Jesus answered and said unto him, If a man love me, he will keep my words: and my Father will love him, and we will come unto him, and make our abode with him.

If one is to have a resulting pure heart (Matthew 5:8) with which to see God, it will take time, persistence, and a close relationship with God. There will be much demonic opposition with which to contend (a nuisance but God is much greater and stronger).

Renewing the Mind and Purifying the Heart

There is absolutely no way to develop a mature spirit without renewing the mind and purifying the heart, for it is out of the pure heart that the inner man can really start working. There is also absolutely no way of doing this without attaining a Holy Spirit-taught deep and broad knowledge of the entire Scriptures. To the extent one does not know Scripture, his inner man is blind and deaf.

There is no way to renew the mind without deep and broad knowledge of Scripture, testing all spirits from which one is hearing and which he is releasing in his speech and in his behavior. This testing is and taking all of his thoughts captive in an organized and planned way (2 Corinthians 10:5). The *least* thing spoken of in the Scripture below includes taking thoughts captive.

Luke 16:10

[10] He that is faithful in that which is least is faithful also in much:

and he that is unjust in the least is unjust also in much.

The pathways to spiritual maturity are described below. One must keep going through these cycles constantly. The pathways are interconnected. After doing these spiritual exercises, one will start to discern his own spirit and will also have his mind renewed (more on the direction in which to renew it later); and his heart will be purified. He will be able to start to bless God. Our book *Spirit* has a thorough description with diagrams illustrating these processes of renewing the mind and purifying the heart.

Pathway to renewing the mind

One needs to read Scripture daily (with the Holy Spirit teaching), read through the whole Bible at least annually, and do a lot of extra topic studies. Meditate as you read, and ask God to show you His message in the passages.

Ask God to start developing the senses in your inner man. Make plans to spend more time and energy studying the spiritual realm and how it impacts the natural realm instead of trying to understand the spiritual realm with a natural-realm mindset. It is impossible to suceed in the latter. Plan with God how you can serve Him better; how you can learn to love Him more; and how you can best praise Him, worship Him, and bless Him. One needs to understand Hebrews 1:3 and 11:3 in order to appreciate the magnitude of the difference between the false wisdom, understanding, and knowledge, taught by the world system through our parents, schools, and colleges, and the true wisdom, understanding, and knowledge taught by God. We will look at these two Scriptures in Hebrews in Chapter 4. These false entities stand only until one sees truth, as God performs miracles which challenge them. Turning water into wine turns material science upside down; walking on water shows that laws of flotation are good only in a limited sense; being transfigured destroys time and the natural-realm concept of the structure of man; and parting the sea destroys climate and weather lore. Holding back the Jordan river and stopping the sun from going down show that all of the descriptors of physics, mechanics, quantum mechanics, and material science hold true only in the absence of a specific spiritual force. Even today we have known people used by God to raise people from death; we have seen major storms rerouted; and we have experienced rain being held off. Renewing the mind involves focusing on the reality of the spiritual realm and its superiority in all aspects over the natural-realm structure and function.

God is so powerful that He can cause atoms to form from subatomic particles, and He can keep them stable; and He can do all of these processes billions of times over within mere seconds. If one has any knowledge of particle physics he will understand the energy involved in doing this even occasionally.

There are four steps to take to renew our mind after we contemplate the above facts so that we have an overall idea of where our mind is now and where it needs to be. We have to change completely from being natural realm focused and from using natural-realm facts and reasoning to being spiritual realm focused and using spiritual-realm facts and reasoning.

We must also understand that the spiritual and the natural realms surround each other and are intertwined (as the mountains surround Jerusalem so God surrounds His people [Psalm 125:2]). We will discuss the related example of the vision given to Elisha's servant (2 Kings 6:17-18) in Chapter 4.

The four steps in renewing the mind within this overall context are (we are assuming one has been through the second birth as this is a prerequisite to renewing the mind):

1. Examine each thought coming into your mind to see if it is coming from the inner man, in which case you should accept it and act on it. If it is not, then it is coming from your flesh, your soul, your heart, or an evil spirit. In any of

the latter cases reject the thought, and do not act on it. It is very helpful to see the motivation of the thought. We only have two resources to offer to God—our time, which we need to redeem, and our resources. The inner man under the influence of Holy Spirit will not waste our time or resources but will maximize these for use by God. Our flesh will try to waste both, and so will evil spirits. Our heart and our soul may do either.

2. Reject or accept the behavior and speech suggested by the thought; and if you have to reject it, repent of the beliefs and attitudes behind it. You can ask God to help in doing better next time.

3. Read the Scriptures, and study them daily, as suggested above. This will increase your sensitivity to God and also will increase your understanding of your motivations and of truth.

4. Continue, taking the next thought captive. When you first starts doing this try to focus on it for one hour twice a day. The process will soon become automatic as you understands your motivations better. It becomes automatic after a few weeks to months, just like driving a car or riding a bicycle. As you talk with God about your thoughts and as you study His Word under the Holy Spirit, you will start to hear Him speaking with you. As time passes it will become easier to discern His voice and communications to you. As you also contemplate all that occurs to us (1 Thessalonians 5:18) and capture these events, you will see better what God is doing to train you.

Purifying the Heart

We purify our hearts through faith.

Acts 15:9

⁹ And put no difference between us and them, purifying their hearts by faith.

Purifying our hearts involves another cycle. When we understand a thought from God asking us to perform a task and when we believe God and perform the task, we start to see that we can trust God when He speaks to us.

This trust builds up from small to big things over time and leads us to trust God when He speaks to us. We are also able to recognize better when God is speaking to us. As we continue to perform the work of God, He will trust us with more; and the whole process increases to the point at which we are able to accept all of the Scriptures as truth. We see God's character more clearly. By increasing obedience to God we allow Him to get rid of the unwholesome and evil buildings in our heart, to remove the slime, and then to start laying foundations and building structures based on the truth in His Word. This whole process leads to purification of our heart.

As our hearts are being purified, we will have just good imaginations and desires, and we will daily mortify the flesh. We can expect to see God, at least in the spirit, at that point so that the Scripture will not be broken (Matthew 5:8).

Our hearts will be reasonably pure when we can always discern God, when we are always obedient to Him, and when we always love God.

We have looked at a lot of God's character traits, and we will now look at His intellect and His power. We will do this in Chapter 4, since both are in need of careful understanding.

God's Character shown in His Intellect and Power

Chapter Four

God's Intellect

One of the most impressive examples of God's intellect is the one we mentioned in Chapter 3 about God's ability to decide between many outcomes in history and to make a choice which would give Him the most pleasure.

Luke 10:13

[13] Woe unto thee, Chorazin! woe unto thee, Bethsaida! for if the mighty works had been done in Tyre and Sidon, which have been done in you, they had a great while ago repented, sitting in sack-cloth and ashes.

In this Scripture God shows that He can foresee all that could oc-cur even in a few small towns over a short time period. Perhaps even more spectacular is that He made man with an ability to choose freely his own destiny for eternity. However, the choices are only two-fold—eternity with God or eternity without being in the presence of God. He does not coerce or manipulate anyone, but He does let each person know the consequence of his choices.

Other examples of His intellect are the variety and design of all of the parts of the creation and how they all interact. There is great variety in the flora and fauna. There is great beauty in music and art. He made man in His own likeness (image) and gave him an environment where he could be creative. Seeing His people being creative is pleasing to Him. Of course, man cannot create anything outside the created spiritual and natural realms; for this is beyond the limit of his abilities. Men have built machines and computers but nothing approaching even remotely to the creation of man. Some of what man has created has beeen given to indi-vidual inventors by spirit beings. God, a spirit, showed Moses the pattern for the Tabernacle in the heavens. A man given something by an evil spirit is likely unaware of the origin of the thought, which he may attribute to his own imagination.

Other examples which show God's intellect include His awareness of a sparrow dying (falling to the ground); knowing the number of hairs on a man's head; and His planning a work for each of His children before the foundation of the world and guiding each person into that choice. God announces events thousands of years ahead of their occurrence. The future of this creation will end just as predicted in the book of The Revelation.

God knows everything in the heart, all of the thoughts, and all of the acts of everyone who has ever been alive or who is yet to be born. Before Esau and Jacob were born God named them and knew what each would do in life, stating, "Jacob have I loved but Esau have I hated." He knows our developing bodies in the womb and before this had designed our features (Psalm 139).

God has plans for all men before they are even conceived. His first command to man was to be fruitful and multiply. When men interfere with this plan through abortions and with other devices, they are bringing down a judgment on themselves; for they are directly interfering with the eternal plans of God.

Genesis 1:28

[28] And God blessed them, and God said unto them, Be fruitful, and multiply, and replenish the earth, and subdue it: and have dominion over the fish of the sea, and over the fowl of the air, and over every living thing that moveth upon the earth.

Romans 9:13

[13] As it is written, Jacob have I loved, but Esau have I hated.

Psalm 139:16

[16] Thine eyes did see my substance, yet being unperfect; and in thy book all *my members* were written, *which* in continuance were

fashioned, when *as yet there was* none of them.

God will judge everyone who who does not go through the second birth at the great white throne judgment at the end of the age. His judgment will include reviewing all of the thoughts and actions a person had and did throughout his life; he is judged by his works. Many events in the Old Covenant pointed to the advent and the work of the Lord Jesus Christ. The first Passover, celebrated in Egypt before Moses led the people of Israel out of Egypt, in the Exodus shows many details of the crucifixion, even down to the placing of the blood on the door posts resembling a cross. If a person has accepted the Lord Jesus Christ as his Lord and as his Savior, then God will count this man as righteous and will accept him as an adopted son. he will not be judged at the great white throne judgment.

Isaiah 66:18

[18] For I *know* their works and their thoughts: it shall come, that I will gather all nations and tongues; and they shall come, and see my glory.

God's intellect allows Him to recall every thought and every action that every person has ever had or made. He will use these facts at the great white throne judgment at the end of this age.

Revelation 20:12–15

[12] And I saw the dead, small and great, stand before God; and the books were opened: and another book was opened, which is *the book* of life: and the dead were judged out of those things which were written in the books, according to their works. [13] And the sea gave up the dead which were in it; and death and hell delivered up the dead which were in them: and they were judged every man according to their works. [14] And death and hell were cast into the lake of fire. This is the second death. [15] And whosoever was not found written in the book of life was cast into the lake of fire.

Be careful to believe the Biblical account.

If one doubts the Biblical account, he has to explain well-observed miracles in the past and present; in addition he has to explain prophesy which has been accurate over thousands of years; and he has to explain the fact that many people have come to know God personally with the result that their lives have been turned around 180 degrees in a very short time. In general, those who doubt the validity of the Scriptures have never studied them in any detail. They mostly echo or parrot a so-called "authority."

When one meets the living God, the truth of the Scriptures and the accuracy of the Scriptures gradually are built as structures in his heart forever. People come to love God. What makes this confusing for an outside observer is that many who think that they have been through the second birth actually have not done so. There are tests one can apply (1 John 5:13) to see if he has been through the second birth. Some people are uncertain about this; and the evil spirits will try to confuse a person who has been through the second birth and will try to make him doubt the reality. People can be very self-deceived about their eternal destination and all should consider the following Scripture carefully:

Matthew 7:22–23

[22] Many will say to me in that day, Lord, Lord, have we not prophesied in thy name? and in thy name have cast out devils? and in thy name done many wonderful works? [23] And then will I profess unto them, I never knew you: depart from me, ye that work iniquity.

God's Power

If we ask individuals what they consider to be great displays of power, the list would probably include earthquakes, volcanic eruptions, nuclear explosions, and even nuclear fusion (which has never been able to be sustained by man). Possibly hurricanes, tsunamis, and other violent storms would be on the list.

God tells us several things which are quite astounding in His Word about His power. Two very important ones occur in Hebrews 1:3 and in Hebrews 11:3. We will also look at the healing of the centurion's servant by the Lord Jesus through the delegating of and sending His spiritual servants (Matthew 8:8-13).

We are also going to look at the control God has of the creation at a subatomic level with the turning of water into wine and at the macroscopic astronomical level with the holding back of the sun. In addition, we will consider the feat of Elijah in causing rain after a drought, the walking on water of the Lord Jesus and the apostle Peter, and the healing of the blind man in two phases.

The display of God's power is exciting to us. It is one thing to be asked to trust a miracle without any notion of how it was performed; but it becomes much easier, we think, when one can see a little glimpse into the mechanics of how it was performed. God has given Bruce a small degree of understanding about how He uses His power in the supernatural realm and also in the natural realm.

We begin by looking at Hebrews 1:3 and 11:3.

Hebrews 1:3

³ Who [Jesus] being the brightness of *his* glory, and the express image of his person, and upholding all things by the word of his power, when he had by himself purged our sins, sat down on the right hand of the Majesty on high.

Hebrews 11:3

³ Through faith we understand that the worlds were framed by the word of God, so that things which are seen were not made of things which do appear.

Bruce asked God about verse 11:3. The answer was for him to consider that a crystal glass can being broken by the right singing pitch and frequency. It seemed that God was implying that

His voice has such power (there are many Scriptures attesting to this) that, by modulating the power, He could form that which appears from spiritual precursors which do not appear. He was able to form subatomic particles and then atoms, molecules, and subsequently large scale matter by the power in His speech. Not only could He do this, but He did it all over the course of six days when He formed the whole natural and spiritual realms. Physicists know the power held in atomic nuclei; in fact, this knowledge led to the development of nuclear devices. God was able to hold atomic nuclei together using spiritual energy in order to form the components of the natural realm. We suspect that these spiritual forces and particles account for the dark matter in the creation that is described by physicists and astronomers. These spiritual-realm components are invisible to the natural realm, but their impact is seen in the natural realm; just as the wind is invisible but the impact is seen in such things as moving trees.

Hebrews 1:3 describes the creation being maintained by continual speech (*rhema*). The original language in this verse indicates that the utterances are continuous. It is this spiritual power in God that created and maintains the functioning of the creation. It cannot be measured by natural devices, since these are all made to extend the range of the natural senses. Without having usable spiritual senses, one cannot understand any more about the spiritual realm's role of maintaining the natural realm within the creation. When man tries to meddle with the atomic nucleus that it is very amateurish and poorly controlled. God can perform microscopic changes and large scale macroscopic changes virtually instantly and without any harm to neighboring structures and people. Such are His power and His intellect.

A person may want to know what evidence there is for this spiritual power operating now and in history. The answer is that this power is the reason for all of the miracles performed by supernatural means. When the United States dropped a nuclear weapon on Hiroshima, the Japanese leaders assumed that it was a sole effort. Three days later Nagasaki was destroyed. In a similar vein the Scriptures record thousands of small and large scale miracles to show that God precisely controls both the natural and the spiritual realms. There is much evidence in history of some major events such as the long day and the long night in the history of various countries. This long day or night accords with the miracle described in the book of Joshua. It is recorded in many historical accounts around the globe (*The Ancient Book of Jasher*). God still performs these miracles. If one is not looking for the hand of God in daily events, he will miss present-day supernatural events. He might call them chance; or he might not deal with them at all if his heart is hardened. We have personally seen God provide for our financial needs by provisions that He made many years ahead. We were unaware of these provisions until the situation arose.

Joshua 10:13

[13] And the sun stood still, and the moon stayed, until the people had avenged themselves upon their enemies. *Is* not this written in the book of Jasher? So the sun stood still in the midst of heaven, and hasted not to go down about a whole day.

The only defense natural man can make to the miracles is to try to persuade people that they did not occur. That will not work with the many people who have received miraculous healings or provisions which were planned years ahead. In fact, we have to realize that the so-called natural laws of physics, mechanics, and quantum mechanics hold most of the time; but they all break down with any miraculous act of God. similar miraculous acts are occuring in current days. God does have stability for people most of the time so that such natural laws do generally hold over long periods of time. We suspect this stability is part of His allowing men to make non-coerced decisions about their future choices. There is a very delicate balance of how much power He reveals. Too much display of power would be coercing to many people; and the absence of, or very limited, displays of power would not raise many people to ask searching questions about their own experiences.

If man could somehow make the sun stand still then the sudden changes in rotation would launch people into orbit. God did it so precisely that this did not occur. He spoke to the elements involved in a perfectly coordinated fashion and all played their role around the globe and out into the solar system and beyond. Only an incredible intellect and power could make such controlled and finely coordinated actions on the creation.

Spiritual Realm and Natural Realm Pairing

There is much in the Scriptures to show pairing of geographic structures in the natural and the spiritual realms. We cannot state whether this pairing occurs throughout the whole creation; but it seems this is case as far as the earth is concerned. 2 Kings 6:8-22 shows that Elisha's servant saw the physical and the spiritual realms superimposed. They appeared as one, but layered on each other.

2 Kings 6:17

[17] And Elisha prayed, and said, LORD, I pray thee, open his eyes, that he may see. And the LORD opened the eyes of the young man; and he saw: and, behold, the mountain *was* full of horses and chariots of fire round about Elisha.

At one point when the Pharisees were complaining about men praising he Lord Jesus Christ He said the following:

Luke 19:40

[40] And he answered and said unto them, I tell you that, if these should hold their peace, the stones would immediately cry out.

We assert that this statement should be believed as literal; it indicates that in the spiritual realm even stones can respond to God with speech. In fact, it seems that the whole universe speaks to the spirit. When a painting or a poem speaks to something within the depth of an individual, this is a spiritual communication. When one is birthed into the spiritual realm, he should experience the whole creation speaking to him about the Lord God and the Lord God's plans. 1 Thessalonians 5:18 illustrates how God expects a person to respond to this communication.

Psalm 19:1–3

[1] The heavens declare the glory of God; and the firmament sheweth his handywork. [2] Day unto day uttereth speech, and night unto night sheweth knowledge. [3] *There is* no speech nor language, *where* their voice is not heard.

Some people would might say that this scripture is metaphorical; but there is no evidence that this is the case, and there is much evidence in the overall context of God's power and His descriptions of the spiritual realm to understand it as a plain statement of fact, as was the statement about the stones crying out.

Men before the second birth have a spirit that is still functional but it is cut off from the life of God. The spirit in a man can perceive some of the spiritual speech of the natural realm, but the person may not hear it with his natural hearing. Nevertheless it is *heard* by the person. There are many types of voices in the world, the dead spirit hears some of them better than others. Music is a language which is heard better in the spirit than spoken languages. It is also more universal in the way people understand and interpret it, so that it can unite spirits. Evil spirits also use music to speak to their followers. God's Word shows that death in the spirit is separation from the life-giving Spirit of God. 1 Corinthians 14:10 points to the great diversity of speech types in the creation.

1 Corinthians 14:10

[10] There are, it may be, so many kinds of voices in the world, and none of them *is* without signification.

The power of evil spirits

It is worthwhile to mention the power of demonic forces at this point. The evil angels have great power compared with men.

However, compared with God they are quite limited; and it would be worthwhile reviewing two accounts. First in Job 1, the discussion between Satan and God shows that Satan cannot go beyond boundaries set by God. Secondly, Exodus 8:1-19 shows that Pharaoh's magicians could manage to perform only the first three miracles. They could not bring out lice and said to Pharaoh that the miracles performed by Moses showed the finger of God. Satanic power flowing into man can perform a limited number of miracles; but after the limit God triumphs. Of course Satan is a created angel.

Other miracles to consider in order to understand the power of God

Elijah's bringing up rain after a prolonged drought showed God's control over the weather. We should be careful to note that God uses local weather changes to bring rebuke to nations and geographic areas, but we need to be careful in attributing weather-related issues to political issues, since not all weather changes are specially ordained by God for rebuke. However, some are, and it may be difficult to know which changes are specially sent by God for His purposes. Consider also the power God placed into the spirit in Elijah which made him able to run ahead of King Ahab who was in a chariot with horses. See the Scripture below from 1 Kings 18:46. God sometimes gives power to the spirit in a man which allows "superhuman" feats. There are many examples of this. Sampson's strength is one example; the miraculous recovery of the Apostle Paul from being stoned is another. The transportation of Philip in the spirit to speak with the Ethiopian man is another (Acts 8:26-40).

1 Kings 18:46

[46] And the hand of the LORD was on Elijah; and he girded up his loins, and ran before Ahab to the entrance of Jezreel.

Turning water into wine

The miracle of Jesus' turning water into wine was well observed by several people. This miracle could not be replicated in the natural realm; spiritual realm-intervention (in this case from God) effected the result that was seen in the natural realm. It is interesting to note that the alchemists in the past tried to turn mercury into gold. They used occult practices (this is demonic spiritual power and not God's power) and it is evident from the miracle that transformations of one material to another can be done by using spiritual-realm forces. We have discussed above how God could modulate the energy in His voice to allow subatomic particles to coalesce into larger atoms, molecules (Hebrews 11:3); and then larger aggregates of matter. All of this was done during the creation very rapidly in billions of places, and now spiritual forces are used to keep the resulting structures intact (Hebrews 1:3). These structures are maintained by spiritual forces which cannot be accessed in the natural realm. The impact of these spiritual forces is similar to the example that we have used with the wind. We see the effects of wind (as in trees blowing) but we do not see the wind itself. What the Lord Jesus Christ probably did was to speak to the water and change it into another substance (wine) in a manner similar to the process used in the creation. He would either have to have moved the elements of the wine from one part of the spiritual realm to another or to have created a new set of elements in the spiritual realm. Either feat is possible using the great powers available in the spiritual realm. Using spiritual forces does not disturb the rest of the natural realm, because these spiritual forces only impact specific spiritual realm receptors. These receptors are able to accept a spiritual realm force only. Thus, just as with the sun staying still with no other apparent impact, the water is turned into wine. The Lord Jesus after the resurrection showed the reality of spiritual forces and specific receptors when He could move through material substances readily. Doors were not a barrier to Him. A natural realm example of specific forces and receptors. is seen with magnetic forces. If one holds a magnet above a non-magnetizable pellet nothing happens.

On the other hand if one holds the magnet above magnetizable metal the small pellet will be picked up by the magnet because it has "receptors" which respond to magnetic force. It is not surprising that the natural realm has only very special receptors for spiritual realm forces which are only discernible to, and usable by, higher-level spiritual beings.

The miracle of turning water into wine and other miracles show man that he is in a natural realm, which is a small training ground in which he is to learn spiritual wisdom, understanding, and knowledge while growing in the family of the Lord God. After receiving the second birth, one has to think in terms of the spiritual realm and learn about operating in it to be pleasing to God. He alone can arrange and supervise our training in the spiritual realm. As one learns spiritual realm precepts, he is able to be much more effective as a tool for God to use in the natural realm.

The healing of Lazarus

Perhaps one of the greatest healing miracles performed by the Lord Jesus Christ was that of Lazarus, whose flesh had been dead four days. Many chemical processes had to be reversed—the deterioration of brain tissue and the breakdown of cardiac muscle, among many other changes. All were reversed within a few seconds, as the creative power in the Lord's voice quickly performed all of the molecular changes in all of the cells, repaired broken cell walls, restarted all of the biochemistry as if nothing had occurred, and restored intellect consistent with the lost time. This shows both the great power of the Lord Jesus Christ over natural realm-matter and His incredible intellect to make all of these changes very rapidly and without any disturbance to the surrounding people and other natural structures. God has established a hierarchy of angelic powers under Him, and He delegates much of this work of restoration and healing to them. Some angels are possibly quite small and similar to the microscopic level in the natural realm. In a miracle such as the healing of Lazarus we could envisage a small army of spiritual beings working under the direction of the

Lord Jesus Christ as he spoke to Lazarus. The miracle done for the centurion shows that the Lord Jesus Christ delegates to angels some of His works.

Matthew 8:8–9

[8] The centurion answered and said, Lord, I am not worthy that thou shouldest come under my roof: but speak the word only, and my servant shall be healed. [9] For I am a man under authority, having soldiers under me: and I say to this *man*, Go, and he goeth; and to another, Come, and he cometh; and to my servant, Do this, and he doeth *it*.

The miracle shown below is fascinating for it contains a more significant miracle within it, as do other healings, which one does not tend to think about in a casual reading. We will take a closer look.

Mark 8:23–25

[23] And he took the blind man by the hand, and led him out of the town; and when he had spit on his eyes, and put his hands upon him, he asked him if he saw ought. [24] And he looked up, and said, I see men as trees, walking. [25] After that he put *his* hands again upon his eyes, and made him look up: and he was restored, and saw every man clearly.

This miracle and all of the healing miracles contain a second and more incredible spiritual deed. One can assume that this man was born blind (others were, if not this man). If a surgeon removed a congenital cataract (*congenital* means "present at birth") from each eye, the individual would have light hitting his retina but he would have to be taught then how to recognize the patterns in order to make sense of the experience; in essence, he would need to learn to see.

After the Lord touched this man's eyes a second time he could see normally. In the other healing miracles the restored limbs, the decomposed bodies of those raised from death, and other events brought each person to a balanced restoration where they were functional at an appropriate level without the need for rehabilitative physical therapy, occupational therapy, and such treatments. The deaf and dumb could speak normally and hear language normally so that their knowledge was restored instantly at the time mechanical and neurological control of speech and hearing were restored. Peter's mother-in-law did not need the usual convalesence after being healed by the Lord Jesus Christ from a fever (Mark 1:30-31).

The Transcendence of the Spiritual Realm over the Natural Realm

The spiritual body does not obey natural laws. The Lord Jesus Christ was given the spirit without measure; and the power in His Spirit could bring healing, and it allowed Him to walk on water. After His death He also demonstrated that His Spirit could teleport Him into rooms without going through doors. The evangelist Philip was transported by the Spirit after baptizing an Ethiopian leader (Acts 8:39).

The supernatural realm is the place to start when one wishes to discern truth. Beacuse all of the laws of the spiritual realm functiong and time are different from those in the natural realm, one cannot reason from the laws of and events in the natural realm to understand the spiritual realm. In order to understand the spiritual realm,, one must have senses developed to see and hear in it. One can reason from the laws of the spiritual realm to explain natural realm situations. When one is reasoning and thinking, it is wise to keep in mind that the thoughts of other individuals are transparent, to an extent, to demonic spirits in both realms. Thoughts can be subjected to deceit in the natural realm when dealing with other people because of the two sets of senses. The Scriptures describe many spiritual laws. A lot of them are based on relationship and the emotions associated with it. Trust in God and holding beliefs in one's heart for God's Words are very important for a person to be able to act in the spiritual realm. Mark 11:23-24 speaks very clearly about this.

Mark 11:23–24

[23] For verily I say unto you, That whosoever shall say unto this mountain, Be thou removed, and be thou cast into the sea; and shall not doubt in his heart, but shall believe that those things which he saith shall come to pass; he shall have whatsoever he saith. [24] Therefore I say unto you, What things soever ye desire, when ye pray, believe that ye receive *them*, and ye shall have *them*.

Conclusion

In the last two chapters we have covered some of the attributes of God's power, His emotions, and His intellect.

We have a glorious God who has plans to prosper us and not to harm us. He brings us to the spiritual realm as a child through a second birth. We can be curious; we can be imaginative; but mostly we can be ebullient relating to our heavenly Father who wants this relationship and who desires to raise up a family for the future ages. As we look at what lies ahead for us, we can only look up and praise the Lord God for great things He has done.

After the second birth God with His power and His intellect arranges that all things work together for good for His adopted children (and for those who do not want to be adopted, He underwrites their decision and gives them what they want). The two scriptures below are very worth contemplation.

Romans 8:28

[28] And we know that all things work together for good to them that love God, to them who are the called according to *his* purpose.

Proverbs 16:9

[9] A man's heart deviseth his way: but the LORD directeth his steps.

Proverbs 16:9 is indeed a powerful Scripture. It shows that God can arrange to have all men walk in the way that they have chosen by arranging circumstances to allow this. He is doing this for five billion or more people daily at this point in history. If a person chooses to come to God that will occur; if he choose to go away from God He will arrange that for him. All of this happens in the background of the daily activities of everyone and is not intrusive. It is awe inspiring and frightening if one chooses against God. God will try to work with those who choose against Him to a point; but His Spirit will not always strive with them, and only God knows this point for each person.

If a person has been through the second birth and loves God (not many do) and is prepared to be obedient to Him (three pre-conditions), then God will make all things work together for that person's good.

God does have the power and willingness to heal.

It should be very obvious now that God is well able to heal and that He is willing to heal. It is very worthwhile for any person who desires God to heal him to ask God for this. He is kind, merciful, and generous. One has to believe that God is who He is. We have to recall that God is working multiple things in the lives of billions of people and that His healing will not necessarily come at the time we want it. We may have to be patient. God will sometimes test this aspect of our character to improve it. When we want healing (and perhaps are in pain), then we tend to be single-focused; but God has to manage billions of tasks and coordinate them all. We must remember that for Him to raise someone from death is no greater effort than to heal, so we must not be driven by fear while waiting for healing. We must keep in mind God's character when we are waiting; He will not harm anyone who seeks Him. In fact, the devil and our flesh can discourage us if we have our focus in the natural realm and have a poorly-developed spirit. Being mature and being strong in the spirit help when we are waiting for God's time.

Proverbs 18:14

[14] The spirit of a man will sustain his infirmity; but a wounded spirit who can bear?

Sometimes we have been healed quickly, and other times have had to wait. God has let us know that we have to wait and that He has heard our request. He told Bruce on one occasion that "God doeth all things well" (Mark 7:37), and Bruce is still waiting for that request to be filled.

we have found that being in God's presence will sometimes expedite healing. In emergencies we tend to use this approach. One has to pray with a combination of spiritual and natural language and seek God to bring him into His presence. One should ask God to fill his spirit with power, peace, joy, and love. We should keep praying until one senses the presence of the Holy Spirit palpably—with alertness, freshness, power, peace, and joy.

We can ask Him to bring us into His presence. This is achieved by coming into His gates with thanksgiving in our heart and entering His courts with praise. Many people do this, but one may still want to get God's attention above the crowd. The Scripture below shows that two people of the many who were in the Lord's presence got His attention.

Matthew 20:29-31

[30] And, behold, two blind men sitting by the way side, when they heard that Jesus passed by, cried out, saying, Have mercy on us, O Lord, *thou* Son of David.

When we can be in a situation to bring blessing to God, we will indeed be in His presence. We have to persist and keep asking, seeking, and knocking (Luke 11:9) when we want something from God. We also have to believe in our heart (see discussion in subsequent chapters) heart to increase his chances of being healed.

The first time Bruce was healed, he did not know much about any of these things we have just written. God healed out of His mercy and initiated the encounter. Subsequently, Bruce has studied healing by God intensively and has been able to build structures in his heart to be able to deal with health issues. These consist of a lot of Scripture passages built into a more global understanding of God and healing. He understands that God is always willing to heal unless there is a blockage. Evil spirits at many levels will try to block people from being healed; and one's own sin can block it.   Evil spirits do not like people's being healed since healing is a powerful sign to the un-saved; they also will try to steal it when it does occur. We will look at factors which block healing in Chapter 7.

Next Chapters

In Chapter 5 we will take a brief look at how God has made the spiritual man. In all ways it is important to have a thorough grasp and understanding of this, since the natural flesh was made to support the spiritual man, not the other way around.

We will look in Chapter 6 at those conditions which increase the likelihood that God will heal and those situations which make it less likely that He will. We will talk about the power of the flesh and the power of evil spirits.

In Chapter 7 we will look at the enemies of healing and will look at those things which might block God from healing a person.

The Structure and Functioning of Spiritual Man (and the two Realms)

Chapter Five

Introduction

It is very important to understand the structure and functioning of spiritual man when we seek God's healing of our flesh and our spirit or even just our flesh. It is essential to understand it in order to cooperate with God in working with Him toward spiritual maturation. In the natural realm, if a person wished to become stronger, he would have to work out with certain muscle groups; and he would have to eat an appropriate diet. He would also have to do some cardiac and respiratory exercises. A person usually has a good understanding of how his body works and functions in the natural realm. For example, he knows how to get food to provide energy. He knows that he has to keep his eyes open; when he sees something new to him, he has to be educated about the object. All of this knowledge was obtained gradually through education from a number of people. Similarly, in the case of strengthening the inner man and helping God to mature the inner man one must understand how the following parts of the spiritual man's anatomy work together: the spirit, the heart, the mind, the soul, the flesh, the will, and the conscience.

At the close of the last chapter we looked at a Scripture shown again below. We are going to look closely at the relationship between our spirit (inner man) and our flesh, which is modified by the condition and content of our spiritual heart. Below are some Scriptures which we want to examine closely to see why it is so important to understand the content of this chapter so that a person can work with God to position himself for spiritual and physical healing. God in the past has give physical healing without requiring any spiritual healing; and since He never changes, He will continue to do this on occasion. A person given this by God would have to come to Him and believe in his heart that He is willing and able to provide the healing. Such a person would never be able to maintain the healing for very long, since he could not weather the assaults from evil spirits to bring back a situation that could be worse than he had before.

Interactions between the flesh and the spirit (inner man)

Proverbs 18:14

14 The spirit of a man will sustain his infirmity; but a wounded spirit who can bear?

This shows that the condition of the inner man has a strong impact on how well a person can sustain an infirmity over a period of time.

Daniel 4:16

16 Let his heart be changed from man's, and let a beast's heart be given unto him; and let seven times pass over him.

This Scripture shows how important the structures and the landscape one maintains in his spiritual heart are. They will determine one's physical appearance. They will impact how quickly he ages. They will determine his resistance to disease. They will impact his lifespan. There are multiple other outcomes related to the content of the spiritual heart. We have just named a few.

Daniel 4:33

33 The same hour was the thing fulfilled upon Nebuchadnezzar: and he was driven from men, and did eat grass as oxen, and his body was wet with the dew of heaven, till his hairs were grown like eagles' *feathers*, and his nails like birds' *claws*.

This Scripture shows that the type of spiritual heart one has actually impacts the flesh in a very substantial manner.

It is very important for one to have a Scriptural knowledge (knowing appropriate Biblical text) of the way his soul works. Without understanding God's Word pertaining to these things one will not attain spiritual maturity; and he will walk his spiritual life in the flesh as the Corinthian believers walked. This is not pleasing to God.

One other fundamental principle that one must understand is that spiritual maturity will come only from a very close relationship with God and a thorough knowledge of His Word. One must determine to make knowing God the main thrust of his energy and use of time. All other things are going to fade away. It is important to set eternity in one's heart and to lay up treasures in heaven (Matthew 6:20)..

As one understands the issues in this chapter, he will start to lay a foundation which can be further built upon, using resources in our previous books *How to be Led by the Spirit of God: Maturing in the Spirit* and *Spirit*. Both heavily reference Scripture.

The Structure of Spiritual Man

Spirit is unseen with natural vision in the natural realm, but the impact of it is observable.[1] In the spiritual realm and in the natural realm when using spiritual vision one can see spiritual beings. Spiritual beings come in all forms just as natural beings. There are viruses (and spiritual realm equivalents). In addition, there are men and angels in both the natural realm and the spiritual realm.

For this discussion we are going to look just at the spiritual structure of man. The spiritual components of man include:

1. Man has a spiritual heart, which is the core of his being. It follows the outlines of the flesh, but it is not linked to our internal organs in a way that is discernible. It would include all of them in it; but there is no natural realm organ(s) that is equivalent to this spiritual heart, although there are some similarities to the work done by both the natural heart and the spiritual heart.

2. The spirit of man, the inner man, is within the spiritual heart and also follows the outline of the flesh, just as a sword is thrust into a sheath.[2]

3. The flesh is the natural-realm component of the spiritual man and includes all of the muscles, skin, organs, heart, lungs, and brain. It also includes all of the knowledge, ideas, motivations, attitudes, and beliefs which reside in the mind and which are not truth received from God. It and the spirit are always antagonistic to each other. They take opposite sides of any issue. (Galatians 5:17).

4. The soul is the combination of the flesh and the spirit (Genesis 2:7 and Ezekiel 37:9-10). When the spirit leaves a soul dies, as is the case at death of the natural body. The soul is the entity which *is* a person. When we use the word *I*, we are referring to our soul. It makes all of the final decisions regarding what to say and do in response to incoming information from both the natural and the spiritual senses. In our soul we carry the image of God; and in our flesh since the fall of Adam and Eve we carry much of the character of the devil. Before the second birth the devil has the power to rule a man through the flesh. This flesh carries more power than his unredeemed spirit. However, as a soul turns through observational evidence toward God, then God will strengthen that spirit to withstand the devil. After the second birth our new spirit can rule over the flesh. Our new spirit is from God and of God. It is always opposed to the flesh, which has been judged by God, and sentenced to destruction (we return to dust after the death of the flesh).

5. The mind is another part of spiritual man, but the spiritual realm-mind is composed of four separate minds. The overall decision-making mind is in the soul. The flesh, the inner man, and the heart all have independent minds with wills and desires of their own. God has created in each

man a replica in miniature of the battle which goes on in the whole creation between Himself and the devil, Satan. Our four minds communicate with each other through our heart. All messages from one mind to another traverse the heart. This may seem complicated but it is clear in the following analogy. When a person is trying to make a simple decision about what to wear to a store he will consult the weather to see how to clothe the flesh. He might consider what style clothing to wear in order to appear well-clad, if he meets someone he knows. He might consider his mood and dress in a way to uplift it. In these simple things he has consulted the minds of his flesh, heart, and spirit, respectively using the mind of his soul to make the final decision.

6. We have a conscience which is on the outer surface of our spiritual heart. It monitors all suggestions for action which are sent to the mind of the soul from the heart. This is a response to all events coming into our soul through the spiritual and the natural senses. The conscience sends a message to the mind of the soul regarding any contemplated action which might violate the standards maintained in the conscience. At that point there would be an internal debate in the mind of the soul regarding what to do in response to new information coming to us from our spirit and from our flesh. The mind of the soul evaluates the suggestions sent from the heart, the conscience, the spirit (through the heart usually), and the flesh (through the heart usually) regarding forming a response to any new information coming to the soul from the natural and from the spiritual realms.

7. The soul, the heart, the flesh, and the spirit all have a "will." This is a center in all four minds of the spiritual man. The will of the flesh will always oppose the will of the spirit. The will is the final area in the respective mind which determines a plan regarding incoming circumstanc-

es and seals it into an irretrievable action. This action may be to do nothing about the information.

A brief look at how the seven areas of the spiritual man interact to make decisions

The above seven areas constitute the spiritual man from the viewpoint of the spiritual realm. We will now look at how information comes into a person and how actions are decided based on this information.

Information comes into a soul by the six senses of both the flesh and the spirit. All of it comes into the spiritual heart. The spiritual heart has an internal arrangement of various structures it has built up from life experiences for handling this incoming information. Over time the heart forms beliefs about objects, people, situations, work, God, and many other "life items." It makes a decision about whether these objects are liked or disliked, thus forming an attitude to each. It stores memories. It compares any information coming in to memory, beliefs, attitudes, and learned expectations regarding possible responses to the information. The spirit and the flesh will weigh in, and the heart formulates a response to all of these variables. The heart then sends its suggestions to the mind of the soul as a recommended action. The conscience may attach a recommendation if it feels that there is a moral component. The soul decides what to do and wills an action. New information that has not been dealt with before will require a more thorough review. This is a vast simplification, but one can get some idea of how these areas interact to maintain himself in communication with his surroundings. A relatively simple example to show how this all works.

The need to buy a pound of butter

A person planning the evening meal for the family will at some point begin to gather ingredients. In this example there is a deadline that he has to meet in order to attend an important evening telephone meeting. He is disturbed to find the meal he is planning is short on a major ingredient, butter.

In this example one child has a birthday and he has been promised that his special request will be served. In this example the man preparing the food has been through the second birth but has no spiritual maturity and a very limited exposure to Bible doctrine. The telephone call is about a new job that seems very desirable and for which the man has been working toward for several months. The new job will offer more income, more prestige, and more power. The man is tired after a long day at work and a stressful drive home.

The man observes with his vision that he is short a pound of butter for the special dessert. This information goes into his heart from the mind of the soul which passes all incoming sensory input to the heart.

The man starts to meditate on the issues. He has faced similar situations and has been able to placate children in the past with the promise of something better in the near future. He could explain that the new job will help the whole family. He could explain to the child that he could not take the time to go to the store and that he would get him the dessert, and more in the near future. He gets approval from the flesh for organizing this to his comfort since he is tired and since the flesh approves of the need for more money, prestige, and power. The spirit has not been exercised very much in the past because this man has been living as a fleshly-motivated believer. He does not think of praying for God's opinion on the decision; he feels that he should not trouble God with what seems to be a minor decision. He feels that it really is not that important and he assumes that God is blessing him with the potential new job.

His heart sends the decision to the mind of his soul along the lines that this has been the way similar situations have worked in the past and that the child may be a little disappointed but that it will do him good to learn to cope with disappointments. There are a lot of high expectations for the whole family with the new job.

Conscience has been blunted over time so that the small voice is felt as a small pang in the soul but is quickly dismissed. The mind of the soul has no spirit-driven counterpoint, since the new spirit is very weak.

The mind of the soul approves all of the fleshly reasoning, and thus the man implements the planned action suggested by the heart. The man chooses a different dessert for the child. He doesn't need to take the trip to the store. The phone call will come at a good time. The will of the soul implments the entire plan.

Hypothetical alternative to the above solution

If the man in the above example is a spirituall-mature individual with a strong history of listening to God and seeking Him in all circumstances (1 Thessalonians 5:18), the results would be quite different.

The pound of butter would also be missing in this example; but in this scenario the man would be aware that the appeal of the new job for power, prestige, and material gain is highly suspicious, since it appeals to the lusts of the flesh. In this example he would have been questioning God all along to see if it is God's desire for him to have the new job. He has promised his son to have the dessert. After a brief prayer he would feel comfortable and at peace driving to the store, getting the butter, and making the dessert. All of the family are aware that the man expects a phone but they take their time at dinner to celebrate the birthday and the child feels very honored when he understands that his father placed him above all else that evening. The family eats the meal with peace and joy. The presence of the Spirit of God is palpably present.

There are so many other spiritual truths to learn from this and every other event which happens to each of us every day. It is how we handle these situations, before God, which will lead to developing purity of the heart and renewal of the mind.

We will now look at one truth which is very important to understand. As we speak and act we can monitor what we say and do to get a better idea of some of the issues in our spiritual heart which may need to be changed.

Examing the content of the heart

In the structure of spiritual man there are built-in devices which explain the Scripture below:

Luke 6:45

[45] A good man out of the good treasure of his heart bringeth forth that which is good; and an evil man out of the evil treasure of his heart bringeth forth that which is evil: for of the abundance of the heart his mouth speaketh.

There is a link between the content of the heart and the things which a man speaks. A person can deceive the in the short run, but not in the abundance of things spoken.

We should note that the Scriptures tell us that only God is good.[3] Therefore, in the verse above, the man described as good is one who has been adopted and trained by God. The evil man is one who has so far not been adopted and trained by God.

We looked at the spiritual heart in more detail in Chapter 4. We are going to look at the flesh in Chapter 6. We are also going to look at the mind further in Chapter 6. In this chapter we will elaborate on Spirit. Much more detail regarding Spirit can be found in our earlier books.

Spirit and what it is

In this section we ae going to confine ourselves to looking at highly intelligent spirits and the spirit in spoken and written words. The highly intelligent spirits are those of God—the Father, the Son, and the Holy Spirit—angels, demons, and men.

With the exception of God and His angels all spiritual beings are usually confined to a natural-realm concept of time and at any one point in time, however small they are able to transmit only one piece of spiritual information. Spiritual beings are constantly exhaling spiritual energy and inhaling it. Spiritual energy is not limited, in the concept of resource depletion, like natural energy is; and the laws describing natural energy do not describe spiritual energy. Only God the Father and God the Son are life-giving spirits. God the Son maintains the whole creation by continually speaking to it in utterances (Hebrews 1:3). This statement is something that will not be understood readily, by most readers and it will take some time to adjust to it and to believe it in a way that changes decision making in life. It violates everything we have learned from the world system. A similar Scripture is Hebrews 11:3. We have mentioned these two Scriptures in Chapter 4 since they are of great importance in understanding the character and the power of God.

The three components of all communications

The whole creation communicates (speaks, writes, and sends various sensory images [visions, odors, touches]) only through flows (our term) of spiritual communications from one being to others. Even natural-realm communications (spoken with audible voice and seen with physical eyes) are all spiritual. There is no such entity as a natural realm only communication. Any flow of spirit involves three parts (components). These three components will vary in intensity depending on the purpose of the communication. We should note that all communication has a motivation (purpose) for it, and this can be spiritually discerned. The motivation is not necessarily discerned by the natural (fleshly) mind. The three components are independent of each other. They are:

1. Power (energy used to perform work toward fulfilling the motivation)

2. Information, which is the description of what is to be conveyed

3. Emotion which is always transmitted, but is clearly received only by spirits who have developed some degree of maturity in spiritual realm functioning

The information in point 2 above may, if it is from God be in the form of a dream or a picture. Demons can also communicate with pictures and dreams. Man, however, is quite limited in the breadth of ways he can communicate information. God and other spirit beings can give communications using any of the six senses so that a recipient could actually have a sense of odor, an audible or inner voice, and even a taste.

If one pauses to think about this he will realize that even a simple word like *no* can be associated with several spiritual messages. There could be anger as with a parent scolding a child; there could be concern as in a parent protecting a child. *No* could be a simple response with little emotion as in refusing an offer of a piece of pie. There is always a motivation, even in offering one word. In the spiritual realm it is hard or impossible to decieve a spiritually mature individual because he will perceive the emotion transmitted. In the natural realm the emotion transmitted will match the content of the transmitter's heart. That may not match the actual words stated. In that case there is intentional deceit (Psalm 55:21).

God's words always have the power to accomplish His purpose. The power in His words sends off secondary cascading events, since God is able to speak to what man considers inanimate objects such as trees, rocks, and other materials. He can also speak to the stars, planets, sun, a paralyzed limb, a storm, and any part of the creation to conform it to His current purpose. He has great spiritual power; and He delegates it in small amounts to His angels, to His children, and to people in government (Romans 13:1-8).

Isaiah 55:11

[11] So shall my word be that goeth forth out of my mouth: it shall

not return unto me void, but it shall accomplish that which I please, and it shall prosper *in the thing* whereto I sent it.

Conclusions

We now have some basic understanding of the anatomy and of the functioning of the spiritual man.

1. The structure of the spiritual man and how he functions

2. The structure of spirit

3. The source of spiritual power and how God shares this

We will now review more about the two realms in the creation—spiritual and natural.

The Two Realms

In the creation there are two distinct and yet interwoven realms. The natural realm we define to be that which is accessed by the six natural senses—sight, hearing, taste, smell, touch, and sense of position in space. We include that which can be accessed by engineered extensions of these senses. This would include seeing the impact of an atom in a cloud chamber, looking at materials with a scanning electron microscope, and using a large array radio-telescope device to explore the heavens. The spiritual realm we define similarly to be that which can be accessed by a set of six analogous senses which belong to our spiritual inner man. We have already, in prior chapters, looked at the close superimposing of the one realm over the other. These are shown in several of the visions people had and which are recorded in the Scriptures (2 Kings 6:17). We have also discussed the differences in how the natural laws do not pertain to the spiritual realm. The spiritual laws do govern the natural realm. Faith in God works in both realms, and belief in the heart works in both realms. Faith, hope, and love work in both realms.

Superiority of the Spiritual Realm

God and the angels are all spirit beings made of spiritual-realm materials. These beings are not confined by physical barriers made with natural materials. Spiritual beings have senses which work in both the spiritual and the natural realms.

The Lord Jesus showed His superiority over the natural realm in the many miracles which He performed. We have looked at the purposes for the creation and see that the major ones included the creation of a family of children who would mature and rule and reign with God in the ages to come. God will, at the end of this age, come from His present abode and live with men in the New Jerusalem on the new Earth.

Man was created with both spiritual and natural senses. After the original sin, when Adam and Eve were expelled from the Garden of Eden, they lost the ability of their spiritual senses to function to much extent. This was a judgment of God on mankind. These senses can be temporarily stimulated by the proximity of a spirit being who has sufficient power. We see the spiritual evidence for this in the presence of such symbols as a third eye, in the crystal ball of a medium, and in the giving of an internal or external vision by God to a person for His purposes.[1]

After the second birth men are given a new inner man (spirit), which is given with the ability to function in the spiritual realm and to allow our soul to function in the spiritual realm after it is trained properly by God. Our natural senses are trained by our natural parents. If this were not done, we would not be able to make sense of the environment. Our eyes might see a car, but that has to be taught as a pattern attached to the name of that object. Our parents might say "blue" for the color blue and "car" for a car. We learned to see by increasingly sophisticated exposure to many objects (learning is the art of making associations with the light patterns hitting our retinas).

In the same way there is a need for a spiritual parent to teach us how to observe, touch, hear, and taste in the spiritual realm. This is God the Father and His delegated teaching to the Holy Spirit, who is given to indwell the heart of every person at the time he goes through the second birth. We have no other guide for this teaching; and, therefore, we have to learn from God directly. God has appointed teachers in the Church. They can teach facts, but few of them can see what someone else is seeing in the spiritual realm. Therefore, one has to rely on God for most of the teaching. We have to learn to recognize His voice in its many tones and modulations. We have to learn to recognize the spiritual-realm patterns which are stimulating our spiritual retinas. Few people have allowed God to train them in how to hear His speech to them; therefore, God cannot train most people to see. Occasionally, God will sometimes open our spiritual eyes with the gift of a vision—either internal or external. We need seek God for further training. We also need to be grateful to God as He patiently trains us to operate in the spiritual realm.

We know people with prophetic gifting who were trained by other prophets as they were both seeing the same spiritual images; so God does delegate some of this teaching to see and to learn to function in the spiritual realm.

The Order of the Two Realms

The spiritual realm has superiority over the natural realm in power; as we see in the miracles which are actually performed according to spiritual laws and are miraculous only to people who observe them in a natural setting. It also has pre-eminence in the things of God. God rules in the spiritual heavenly, realm.[2] He allowed man first[3] and now the devil, Satan, to rule[4] on the earth. Satan operates in boundaries[5] placed by God for His purposes. A defining Scripture is Hebrews 8:5.

The natural realm contains nothing that is not antecedent in the spiritual realm.[6] There is nothing done in the natural realm that is of eternal worth; everything is vain (*lit.*, empty) unless the work originates in the spiritual realm in and from God.[7]

God asks His people to request that His plans be implemented in the natural realm.[8] He will in general do nothing in the earth without the request or without the desire of at least one of His people.[9]

There are several far-reaching conclusions. A major one is that one cannot look at the events in the natural realm with just natural-realm senses, because he cannot interpret many of them properly with just the natural realm understanding. It is vain to speculate and say such things as that climate change might cause a destructive global warming with wide-spread flooding. Unless this is in God's plan (and it is not), then it will never come to pass. All bounding conditions relating to things pertaining to the earth, the politics on the earth, and the geographic conditions on the earth are determined in the spiritual realm (Psalm 2, and there are many similar Scriptures). It is only as one senses with spiritual senses that one can understand the plans of God.[10]

We should never try to use natural reasoning and conditions to understand the future on the earth or to explain the present or the past. It is only as we use spiritual realm observations and knowledge that we will have any true insight and understanding.

We should never try to interpret the things of the spiritual realm with natural knowledge. It is going in the wrong direction and will yield nothing of substance.

Men through the years have developed various ways of trying to see the future independently of God. For centuries this work was done through mediums, the use of which God condemns. In these current times it is also sometimes through statistics which are a decent tool but still of limited help in short range projections involving limited situations. For long-term predictions over broad areas they become highly error prone.

The clear supremacy in all ways of the spiritual realm

The spiritual realm where God maintains His rule is the controlling domain over all aspects of the natural realm, but this control is mediated and modified in many ways through the people of God and their relationship to God. God keeps the overall plan He has for this age moving forward but within this plan there is room for much modification as His people talk with Him and work for Him under His clear direction.

The ability to learn how to work in the spiritual realm through clearly understood and well developed direct communication with God is the key to God's working His most favored plans. If His people do not do this then He defaults to another plan. We, His people, lose the present-age and future-age blessings we could have had when this occurs.[11]

It does take much time, effort, and devotion to the things of God to be trained by Him directly. One has to place one's focus on putting Him first in all things. He will not use anyone who is double minded about Him and His Kingdom.[12] There is a present-time cost, but a future enormous gain, for those people willing to place God and His Kingdom above all else. Anything we do for God and His Kingdom has to be led by Him, just as an army needs a general to supervise the overall plans. God in any particular work will determine the amount of direct supervision of any individual. This amount will vary from person to person. We must not make presumptions and must not offer any works conceived in our flesh or in our flesh-contaminated thinking.[13]

Scriptures to read in order to see more of God's power and character

Job 1—to see God's power over the demonic powers including the devil, Satan, to whom God gives certain rights

Job 38-41—to see how God expects man to understand Him in the revelation of His power (showing God's control of the creation)

Psalm 94:1-15, esp. v9—to see the false expectations of fallen men

Psalm 18 and Psalm 19—to see more of the power and the character of God

We can learn to work with God.

We have to learn how to operate in the spiritual realm by direct supervision from God, but there are guidelines in the Scriptures which help us to do that. We need to understand some of the basics about what spirit is and the structure of man from a spiritual-realm perspective. We can gain spiritual-realm knowledge as the Holy Spirit teaches us through the Scriptures. This teaching is available to anyone who has been through the second birth and who is seeking God vigorously.

God's plans for the future ages and the requirements He has for His children in this age

As we said earlier, God made the creation for His eternal purposes. The creation of man in His image is a key part of this. He wants people in His family to rule and to reign with Him in the ages to come and to be a family—with some being a bride for the Lord Jesus Christ.

We do not have many specifics about these future ages, but we do have a lot of information. God will live with His people in the New Jerusalem (Revelation 21:2-3). Revelation 21 and 22 give a lot of information about the future. The Scripture below sets up bounding conditions about the future ages.

Matthew 24:35

[35] Heaven and earth shall pass away, but my words shall not pass away.

Even in the future ages the same Scriptures will apply as they do now. These creative words in the Scriptures always accomplish the purposes God speaks them over.

Isaiah 55:11

[11] So shall my word be that goeth forth out of my mouth: it shall not return unto me void, but it shall accomplish that which I please, and it shall prosper *in the thing* whereto I sent it.

The present-age purposes of God for His children

We have mentioned earlier that the present age is a training ground and that God requires a certain type of character in the people that He adopts into His family. The Scripture below presents this idea. God's children need to be undergoing training from Him, as we have indicated in earlier chapters. This is very important for spiritual wellness and healing. Spiritual healing is very important for physical healing.

One should meditate deeply on Ephesians 2:10-22, because it speaks of further purposes of God for His children in this age.

[20] [citizens of God's household] are built upon the foundation of the apostles and prophets, Jesus Christ himself being the chief corner *stone*.

In this age God is building a habitation of which the Lord Jesus Christ is the chief cornerstone and upon which the apostles and prophets build a foundation. God's requirement for other corner stones is that these people be like the Lord Jesus Christ and like the foundation of the apostles and the prophets. We have discussed the mechanisms for how one can bring this about in his life.

1 Corinthians 13:12–14:1

[12] For now we see through a glass, darkly; but then face to face: now I know in part; but then shall I know even as also I am known. [13] And now abideth faith, hope, charity [love], these three; but the greatest of these *is* charity.

These character traits are what God seeks of those He will adopt into His family. He can see ahead of the adoption that these traits potentially can be prominent in His children. The Lord Jesus Christ excelled in all three—faith (hearing God clearly); hope (the blessed assurance of the promised future); and charity, which is love.

The Lord Jesus Christ is the first fruits of those conformed to His Image (Romans 8:29). God wants His children in this age to be conformed to the same character as that of the Lord Jesus Christ.

Bruce has been trying to understand what purpose God has in the future for needing these character traits in His people and why those with a set of character traits that reflect their submission to the demonic forces are unacceptable. While pondering this, he saw some things in the spiritual realm which seem to explain God's reasons. This illustrates why it is so important to a person's spiritual development that he go through the process of renewing his mind and purifying his heart in order to be able to communicate with God and to receive the answers to questions like the ones Bruce had been asking. The answers are not particularly important to the discussion in this book; but the fact is that all of God's children should be asking God questions and having Him answer these questions. Since the answers to Bruce's questions are lengthy, we will sttate only some highlights.

Answer to Bruce's questions

1. We are so used to false wisdom, understanding, and knowledge that it is very hard to adjust to a completely new concept, that of non-depleting resources and energy in the spiritual realm in future ages. Resource and energy depletion occurs in the natural realm where there is a restricted presence of God's life-giving Spirit. We have no reason for assuming that in the future ages there will be any bounding of energy, although it is hard to conceive how this could be. Thus, the evil powers have constrained man to think negatively.

2. The evil spirits try to form a relationship with a man in which they can "drain" energy from the person to use for themselves. We see this in demonically-caused illnesses,

particularly malignancies. Evil is directed toward only three goals—to steal, to kill, and to destroy (John 10:10). People who have not been through the second birth and reconciled with God are slaves of evil and thus have one of these three goals at the base of their behavior. There is no unity of spirit, for they want to destroy each other. It is difficult to think about these things; but God's children have to face this truth or we cannot see the character of God as clearly as we need to. Certainly, there is a great variation in the degrees of degeneration of those people who refuse to reconcile to God. Sometiimes it will be hard to see these three foundational goals (stealing, killing, and destroying) in the external behavior in the natural realm; but in the spirit one can see them. This again illustrates why one has to let God strengthen and mature his spirit, or he will never see these issues clearly with just natural-realm understanding. It is difference in feeling the waves of hatred flowing over a person as he is shown a high-level demonic ruler and reading that the demons hate people. This is why one has to start living in the spiritual realm if he wants to understand the Scriptures (1 Corinthians 2:14).

3. In this age God's children are to learn to abhor all evil as one ponders the purposes of evil spirits. God wants His children to look fully into the face of evil and reject it so deeply that in the future ages they will have no desire ever to rebel against God. God's children are also to be conformed, in this age, to the standards set forth in the Scriptures below. We discussed earlier how to go through this process.

Ephesians 4:13

[13] Till we all come in the unity of the faith, and of the knowledge of the Son of God, unto a perfect man, unto the measure of the stature of the fulness of Christ.

Romans 12:9

[9] *Let* love be without dissimulation. Abhor that which is evil; cleave to that which is good.

4. One needs to consider how God builds His creation and what character traits He values in His Kingdom. Review the Scriptures below.

Galatians 5:22

[22] But the fruit of the Spirit is love, joy, peace, longsuffering, gentleness, goodness, faith,

Romans 14:17

[17] For the kingdom of God is not meat and drink; but righteousness, and peace, and joy in the Holy Ghost.

Colossians 3:15

[15] And let the peace of God rule in your hearts, to the which also ye are called in one body; and be ye thankful.

These all show that God elevates the emotions over the reasoning ability of those people whom He has in His Kingdom. He does not need our ideas in this age, for they are inferior to His. Perhaps in the ages to come as His children mature to the point at which they will rule and reign with Him this will be different, and God will want the thoughts of His children.

One has to ask why God focuses on the emotions above reason. He especially elevates faith, hope, and love. Love is the greatest. Not coincidentally, love is the subject of the First and Second Commandments, which will be present in the ages to come. God wants all of His children to be perfected in love.

1 John 2:5

⁵ But whoso keepeth his word, in him verily is the love of God perfected: hereby know we that we are in him.

All of the Scriptures listed above will also be true in the ages to come. We see the need for these emotions and why God wants to exclude the negative emotions of the evil spirits and those emotions of the people still enslaved to them.

5. The Scripture below indicates the importance of the positive emotion of love. The truth of this Scripture is based on how God designed the forces and structures in the spiritual realm to interact.

Ephesians 4:15–16

¹⁵ But speaking the truth in love, may grow up into him in all things, which is the head, *even* Christ: ¹⁶ From whom the whole body fitly joined together and compacted by that which every joint supplieth, according to the effectual working in the measure of every part, maketh increase of the body unto the edifying of itself in love.

Verse 16 shows that the sum is greater than the parts. Earlier we discussed the reductionist arguments that the whole is no greater than its parts. The positive emotions build up, and the negative emotions tear down.

God has so designed the spiritual realm that it grows on the positive emotions—just as one's spirit matures, strengthens, and grows as it takes in the fruit of the Holy Spirit (Galatians 5:22, listed above). God inhabits those who love and obey Him.

The power in the emotions of God

The emotions of God carry a powerful force with them, since they are spiritual in nature and all flow of spirit has to have a degree of power. In the spiritual realm His emotions cause appropriate growth. We also can bring about growth also in the spiritual-realm structures as we are perfected in love.

Proverbs 11:24

[24] There is that scattereth, and yet increaseth; and *there is* that withholdeth more than is meet, but *it tendeth* to poverty.

This Scripture shows how we also can increase an entity through love. Thus, the positive emotions are actually building the creation in the ages to come; this is the opposite of the natural realm energy sources such as oil which are gradually depleted. The growth receptors on the cells in natural man need a chemical hormone, which is gradually depleted during life. The growth receptors God has designed in the Spiritual realm cause growth with the power of love.

Conclusion

We have given a short summary of the reasons for the choices God made in who and why only certain people would be adopted into His family. These adoptees will be able to function and grow in stature, helping each other in unity and love, during the ages to come—in a realm that is incredibly richer in innovation and diversity than anything we see in the natural realm.

Isaiah 64:4

[4] For since the beginning of the world *men* have not heard, nor perceived by the ear, neither hath the eye seen, O God, beside thee, *what* he hath prepared for him that waiteth for him.

1 Corinthians 2:9

[9] But as it is written, Eye hath not seen, nor ear heard, neither have entered into the heart of man, the things which God hath prepared for them that love him.

Superscripts used in this Chapter

1. 2 Kings 6:17 and many other examples such as the writings in the Revelation of John.

2. Deuteronomy 10:14 and Psalm 115:16

3. Genesis 1:28

4. Matthew 12:26 and John 12:31

5. Job 2:1-7

6. Exodus 25:8-9 and Ecclesiastes 1:9

7. Ecclesiates1:14

8. Matthew 6:10

9. Psalm 115:16

10. John 5:19

11. Esther 4:14

12. James 1:6-8

13. Proverbs 14:12

Getting Healed

Chapter Six

Asking God for Healing

When we want God to heal us to heal us and if we are asking the God who wrote the Bible for healing, we are asking an all-powerful God and an all-knowing God, who knows us intimately. In fact, He knows the depths of our character far better and more accurately than we do. He also knows what we will achieve in the future—to the second and to the smallest tasks. We can bring absolutely nothing to the table. Even Moses would not have been able to say to God, "You owe me this." One has to come before God personally, or through other people praying for him, in order to request healing. If one is requesting God to heal him, then one must have some expectation that God is able to heal and that He is willing to heal.

It is relatively easy to believe in the mind that God is quite able to heal people and that He does heal people; but a large number of people asking God for healing, if really questioned closely, will not have a firm conviction that God will heal them at this point in time of a particular problem. Having a belief in the mind is relatively easy, for this is essentially just a distant intellectual assent to God's power. Having a belief just in the mind, without supporting structures in the heart, would not necessarily stop the Lord God healing one. This issue came up with a father's asking healing for his son from epilepsy. When asking the Lord Jesus Christ to heal his son, he also asked Him to help his unbelief. We do not know why He made His decision to heal when faith in the father was incomplete but no doubt mercy and love were involved. He would have known that the father wanted to believe.

In our experience God does not require an in-depth knowledge of His character before He will heal. He actually initiated healing for Bruce on the first occasion of His healing him. He sometimes will heal those who have no intention of becoming His children because He loves all the people that he has created (whether they become part of His eternal family or not). He is merciful and kind; and He is patient. The problem those who do not know Him and who are not in a relationship with Him face is that when they pray they will have no idea of how to test the spirit which seems to be answering them. Evil spirits can take advantage of one's spiritual blindness and can gain a hold over a person who prays to a god they do not specifically name and of whom they have little or no personal knowledge. In the days of the advent of the Lord Jesus Christ it was easier for those who wanted no part of spiritual healing to request healing of a physical disease directly from the Lord.

What are we asking God to heal?

We have to consider what we want healed. On occasion we have fallen short in our request and have not asked for as much as God might have been willing to give. This always displeases God (2 Kings 13:15-19). One can ask for just physical healing; and one can ask for spiritual healing, including salvation. Most people need both spiritual and physical healing. If we are not an adopted child of God and if we do not seek spiritual healing, then we remain with a spirit separated from the life-giving power of God and which is readily subject to both the flesh and demonic powers.

If we are an adopted child of God but have never matured in our spirit, then our new spirit will still be quite subject to the flesh and to demonic powers. It has potential for growth in power, strength, and wisdom, as one starts to let God teach him how to live in the spiritual realm.

In both of the above situations it is easy for an evil spirit to steal the healing. One will not be able to offer much if any resistance. Therefore, it would be wise to seek salvation and spiritual maturing and growth; if one has salvation then he should seek spiritual maturing and growth along with physical healing.

As one matures and grows in spiritual strength, he will gradually get to a place where he may be able to seek all of the benefits God gives in Psalm 103:1-5; which includes renewal of his youth.

God commands that His adopted children seek Him for healing while stopping to sin in acts of omission or commission.

God's adopted children are commanded to be healed in both the spirit and in the flesh (Hebrews 12:13) for this is glorifying to God. His adopted children actually have to block being healed by maintaining sin patterns in their hearts all of which are displeasing to God. God's children develop illness and infirmity due to a combination of one or more circumstances:

a. One such circumstance involves the outworking of natural realm laws—such as too much caffeine causing an ulcerated stomach or smoking leading to lung cancer.

b. A demonic attack totally unprovoked other than to cause problems for a child of the living God (and certain spirits are skilled in bringing particular illnesses), is another circumstance.

c. Some demonic attacks, however, have a basis given by an individual. These include family illnesses which have never been formally broken in the spiritual realm. If one has never renounced the curse, then he will be subject to attack by a familial spirit. Other attacks may be based on a sin pattern which allows a spirit to accuse the person to God successfully.

d. The Lord God will allow demonic attacks and will place illnesses on people who are His children and who do not learn to listen to His utterances to them and who do not obey His commandments. He does it to gain the attention of an individual. If one is used to good health and suddenly becomes ill, he should examine himself before God.

Deuteronomy 28:15

[15] But it shall come to pass, if thou wilt not hearken unto

the voice of the LORD thy God, to observe to do all his commandments and his statutes which I command thee this day; that all these curses shall come upon thee, and overtake thee.

In this Scripture *hearken* is physically hearing, and *voice* is an audible noise.

e. An infirmity might not be healed until a time to glorify God (the raising of Lazarus [John 11:40-44, and also see John 9:3]).

f. Sometimes the circumstance is a special case, as in the case of Job. God found no evil in Job, but He wanted Job to have a greater understanding of Himself. It allowed Job to grow in spiritual understanding and power, which was a good thing for Job (Romans 5:3 and 2 Thessalonians 1:4).

g. There might be other special purposes as with the Apostle Paul (2 Corinthians 12:7-9). Generally, God will let a person know why he has to suffer. On one occasion God let us know that the recurrent trial we were undergoing over several years would work an eternal weight of glory for God (2 Corinthians 4:17). That was all God said to us about it. Also in these special situations God eventually gives healing.

h. Healing may be delayed for numerous reasons that allow God to work out the appropriate time so that He can do all things to maintain His promise to do all things together for our good (Romans 8:28-30).

i. One special sin pattern needs mentioning because it is a significant present-day problem. That is of taking Communion unworthily. This can cause even a premature death. Those of God's children who do not mature in the spiritual realm have little discernment of how seriously God takes such spiritual-realm offenses (1 Corinthians

11:27-31).

j.   A more general case of not judging ourselves applies to many illnesses in God's children. 1 Corinthians 11:31-32 adresses this. Not judging ourselves regarding whether we are hearing God's utterances and obeying all of His commandments and not learning to communicate with God through listening to Him are probably the most prevalent cause of illnesses in the children of God in the Church in the West.

k.   God will always heal His adopted children unless a child refuses to mature or refuses to repent of all sin patterns (Psalm 25:18 and 1 John 3:22 [below]).

1 John 3:22

[22] And whatsoever we ask, we receive of him, because we keep his commandments, and do those things that are pleasing in his sight.

1 Corinthians 11:31–32

[31] For if we would judge ourselves, we should not be judged. [32] But when we are judged, we are chastened of the Lord, that we should not be condemned with the world.

Faith for healing and the need for spiritual development and maturity

If an adopted child does not have faith in God's provision of healing, then this will likely be a reason that God will not heal. 1 John 3:22 shows the need for a high level of spiritual maturity. When a child of God refuses to mature, God is not pleased (Colossians 1:10 below); but God is God, and He may still choose to heal out of His mercy and goodness. We can never speak for God in any individual situation, since only God knows the content of a person's spiritual heart. The degree of faith in God that one has is directly related to his spiritual maturity and to his purity of heart.

Failure to repent of such issues as not taking thoughts captive, not purifying one's heart, and not renewing one's mind will most likely disqualify him for the blessing of 1 John 3:22. In Hebrews 12 we noted that God commanded healing for His adopted children, but we must be careful to note that this command was in the overall context of removing chastening for our sin patterns so that God will heal.

Colossians 1:10

[10] That ye might walk worthy of the Lord unto all pleasing, being fruitful in every good work, and increasing in the knowledge of God;

This Scripture shows that our actions in doing the work that God desires (not that which we decide but rather a work definitely given by God) well and maturing in our relationship with God are pleasing to Him. Not maturing displeases God. There are very definite steps a person can take to get to know God better (and thus mature). We have discussed these in earlier chapters—renewing his mind, taking his thoughts captive, and purifying his heart.. As we please God, we are likely to be blessing Him and will fall under the provision of Psalm 103:1-5 and 1 John 3:22.

God has given instructions for ways to access healing including those in James 5. Usually there will be a need at the same time for spiritual healing (more patience, more understanding of the spiritual realm through improved vision and hearing, and many other possibilities). God expects those who receive much from Him in terms of talent, instruction, healing, and all other areas of life to give more back to God in terms of volunteered service (Luke 12:48).

Healing for those who are not adopted children of God

God is sometimes willing to heal those who are not His children. Frequently, however, the attitudes and sin patterns in the heart and the geographic area in which one lives prevent a person's being healed (See our earlier book: *Healing*). There will not be a voluntary service requirement for those people who have not been through the second birth. Any healing that God gives such a person would be a gift. God certainly uses those who have not been through the second birth to work His eternal plans, but it is not a form of service to which the individual accedes. Examples of such people being used by God include the King of Assyria and Pharaoh.

Essential Requirements for God to heal an individual

There are no set requirements, although there are ways to increase the likelihood of being healed to near certainty. The son of the widow of Nain (Luke 7:11–14) had met no particular requirements.

[11] And it came to pass the day after, that he went into a city called Nain; and many of his disciples went with him, and much people. [12] Now when he came nigh to the gate of the city, behold, there was a dead man carried out, the only son of his mother, and she was a widow: and much people of the city was with her. [13] And when the Lord saw her, he had compassion on her, and said unto her, Weep not. [14] And he came and touched the bier: and they that bare *him* stood still. And he said, Young man, I say unto thee, Arise.

God is very compassionate. Healing is closely linked to salvation in the Scripture. God provided both in the crucifixion of His Son. Isaiah 53 (in the original language) makes this very clear.

There are many other instances where the Lord Jesus Christ initiated a healing; one other is the man lying beside the pool of Siloam. It is always God who initiates a drawing of someone to salvation; sinful man would not take this step. In a very real sense and in a powerful way it was God who initiated all of the healings during the advent of the Lord Jesus Christ. When people were in the presence of His power and saw and heard at close hand the things that He did, they were drawn to Him. For people to be able to respond to God for salvation and for healing there usually have to be two elements—faith, and belief. God is willing to help with both.

God's Healing Power

God's power is able to accomplish work only when there is something capable of responding to it. God can exert all of the power in the creation to persuade one individual to accept Him as His redeemer; but if there is no receiving element in the heart and mind of that person, then the power will not result in any change. God made all men free to be able to respond to Him or to reject Him. After Adam and Eve sinned in the Garden of Eden, several things happened. Their spirits no longer received regular infusions of the spirit of life from the Spirit of God; their flesh would die and return to dust; and they now knew the difference between good and evil. This knowledge of good and evil is present in the heart of all descendants of Adam and Eve. It is this knowledge of good and evil which allows a person who wishes to be drawn by desiring good to come into a relationship with God. If a person chooses to be drawn by evil, that individual is very unlikely to come into a relationship of any kind with God.

The salvation from the sin nature with which all people are born, the eventual resurrection from the state of physical death, and the healing of illness and infirmity show God's great power to a world that is lost. God uses illness, infirmity, and the act of healing His people as a testimony of His character to those who have not been through the second birth. There are a few times that God healed in the period of His incarnation on earth where the healing was not sought. In almost all cases of healing during the incarnation of the Lord Jesus Christ there was a seeking for the healing. Probably one would not want to depend on God's arbitrarily deciding to heal him, when it is easy to seek Him for healing.

Increasing the likelihood of God's healing a person

Probably one would like to know how best to approach God with a request for healing so that it is very likely to be granted. There are barriers which make healing unlikely, which we listed above; and there are steps we can take to make healing very likely. We can never speak for God in any given situation, and these things which we have written are generalizations. There is nothing better for a person to do than to get to know God and speak with Him one on one when requesting healing.

Healing of physical illnesses is frequently confined to a specific time and to a specific illness or infirmity. It is not permanent, and it can lapse if one starts to doubt as the devil tries to steal the healing. Healing by God is without side effects, and it is given to the child of God to encourage him in his relationship with God. It is an act of mercy and kindness by a loving heavenly Father. Psalm 103 gives a contrast to limited healing. In it there are magnificent promises of healing all of one's diseases and renewing one's youth (*e.g.*, Caleb and Joshua).

Psalm 103:1–5

[1] Bless the LORD, O my soul: and all that is within me, *bless* his holy name. [2] Bless the LORD, O my soul, and forget not all his benefits: [3] Who forgiveth all thine iniquities; who healeth all thy diseases; [4] Who redeemeth thy life from destruction; who crowneth thee with lovingkindness and tender mercies; [5] Who satisfieth thy mouth with good *things; so that* thy youth is renewed like the eagle's.

1 John 3:22 reprinted below. and Colossians 1:10, printed above show that we can please God and bless God by the closeness of our relationship with Him—becoming spiritually mature and performing well the specific commands He gives for work. We also have to fulfill His general commands written in Scripture. If we can fulfill the First Commandment with a true and powerful love for God, placing God's needs above ours (Romans 15:3), as the Lord Jesus Christ did, then we would be well on the way to pleasing God and blessing Him.

1 John 3:22

[22] And whatsoever we ask, we receive of him, because we keep his commandments, and do those things that are pleasing in his sight.

Other scriptures also show situations which please God.

Hebrews 11:5

[5] By faith Enoch was translated that he should not see death; and was not found, because God had translated him: for before his translation he had this testimony, that he pleased God.

We do not know a lot about Enoch, other than he was in a very close relationship with God.

Hebrews 13:15–16

[15] By him therefore let us offer the sacrifice of praise to God continually, that is, the fruit of *our* lips giving thanks to his name. [16] But to do good and to communicate forget not: for with such

sacrifices God is well pleased.

This last Scripture from Hebrews is talking about offering praise to God through the Lord Jesus Christ. It is not a vain repetition type of praising but a specific giving of thanks for His character as He has revealed it to us in the relationship we have with Him. We should be continually praising Him in all of the circumstances of our lives (1 Thessalonians 5:18). This Scripture is not talking about a worship service where we sing some praise songs but rather a lifestyle and communication pattern which gives God glory. God is requesting us to communicate with Him (speak to Him and listen to Him) if we are to please Him.

1 Peter 3:4

[4] But *let it be* the hidden man of the heart, in that which is not corruptible, *even the ornament* of a meek and quiet spirit, which is in

the sight of God of great price.

This Scripture in 1 Peter 3:4, when manifested in one's life, is a blessing to God. He sees it as worth a great price. He will work hard to help one to form such a spirit. In Scripture *meek* is not "weak." Moses had one of the most powerful ministries ever given to a man. God termed him as the meekest man. Meekness is an attitude of one's spirit (inner man) toward God first and also to people with whom he is in contact. It is not weak; it is rather a deliberate choice to yield one's inherent power in favor of another, based on one's knowledge of God or of the other person.

Colossians 3:20

[20] Children, obey *your* parents in all things: for this is well pleasing unto the Lord.

This Scripture states one specific way that a person needs to be obedient to God in order to please Him; but this alone will not make one pleasing to God in an overall sense. Failure to perform this would not be easy to make up in God's eyes, since family relationships are a very important part of His eternal plans in the ages to come.

Something with which God is not well pleased

1 Corinthians 10:5

[5] But with many of them God was not well pleased: for they were overthrown in the wilderness.

This Scripture actually shows the impact of not being pleasing to God. It speaks of the Exodus and the judgment on those children of Israel who murmured against God, who did not listen to His voice, and who did not believe Him. God has not changed, and those of His children who are not obedient will frequently be punished by sickness and early death (1 Corinthians 11:30).

Transitioning from one's present situation to being a blessing to God and pleasing Him

The question is how we go from a situation of having a disease healed to obtaining the promises in Psalm 103:1-5 and in 1 John 3:22. The road is long, and great changes will be necessary if one wishes to obtain such rich blessings from God. We cannot guarantee results since it is only the Lord God who can see into the depths of the heart of any individual. We can state that by following the path to spiritual maturity, one will be very likely to fulfill the requirement that he bless the Lord in Psalm 103:1-2 and that he keep all of the commandments of God in 1 John 3:22. We can also state that his likely reward in the eternal Kingdom will be to be a vessel of gold and to have an elevated position. Even above these eternal situations, that individual will dwell close to the presence of God during this life and in eternity.

Desiring to be in the continual presence of God and being granted this are the greatest rewards any adopted child could obtain. We may think that we want this; but in fact most of us will turn aside from being personally close to God and attempt to work for God using our own plans and devices. We will elevate working for God above seeking to be with God (Luke 10:40-42). Man is obsessed with offering sacrifice of something to God instead of offering himself. Offering anything other than himself will not be pleasing to God, and that alone may will block being in His presence.

Romans 12:1

[1] I beseech you therefore, brethren, by the mercies of God, that ye present your bodies a living sacrifice, holy, acceptable unto God, *which is* your reasonable service.

Issues we need to guard against

1. Our work should flow out of being in His presence. Our work will keep us in God's presence only if it is something He has commanded. He will usually try to perfect

our love for Him before He will trust us with great works for Him. When we attempt to use our time and energy to elevate work we do for God above seeking His presence, then we will miss both since most of our work done like this is initiated in our flesh and as such it is filthy to God (Isaiah 64:6).

2. To stay in God's presence, we must eliminate all fleshly presence from us. God hates the flesh unless it is purified by fire. He judged it in the Garden of Eden and withdrew His life-giving spirit from it so that it is dead now and forever. We must perfect the spiritual walk (Romans 8:14). To approach this, we need God to help us to mortify the body (flesh) daily through the leadership of the Spirit of God; and we need Him to train us in being led by His Spirit. As we do this and as we learn to perfect thanksgiving in our heart, and continually to have praise on our lips, then God will bring us into His presence.

Romans 8:13

[13] For if ye live after the flesh, ye shall die: but if ye through the Spirit do mortify the deeds of the body, ye shall live.

When we live after the flesh and are adopted children of God we will be saved through a fire-like experience; but in this life it will keep us from the life of God. If we are led by the Spirit of God, then we mortify the flesh and have the life of the Spirit of God flowing through us as we do His work.

How being in God's presence brings healing to the spirit and to the flesh

We will review Scripture that shows how the life-giving spirit of God flowing through the Lord Jesus (and us when we are filled with the Spirit and have a pure heart) brings healing to all of our diseases. We bless God by always being in His presence, always fulfilling His purposes, and always following His perfect will. The two miracles below show the power coming from God. No man has very much power unless God gives it to him for his particular work—even civic work, government work, law enforcement, or other secular jobs. All people radiate a degree of power depending on the anointing God has placed on them. This power is delegated by God to the spirit of the person, which is the supplier of all of one's energy. The power a person has enables him to do certain works because this power is associated with certain knowledge and is directed to perform needed tasks. Exodus 36:1-2 is an example of how God does this. God has various tasks which He uses His power to fulfill. Whenever a need from any person, for healing touches God, then He will allow His power to flow to fulfill that need. During the advent of the Lord Jesus Christ a physical touch released His healing power. Now we have to reach out with our spirit (not our flesh) to touch His Spirit. We have to learn and understand how to do this.

We have seen that our inner man dwells in our heart. When a person comes before God with a request for healing, the attitudes and beliefs that he holds in the structures in his heart might block some of the flow of healing power through his heart and out into his flesh. It is not only God who may limit or refuse to give healing power, but we also can do that. If a person's heart has been purified through faith, then the healing power of God can flow straight through the heart and into the flesh. Of course, God may choose not to heal any person at a specific time for a greater work that He is performing over a wider area and involving more people.

Matthew 14:35–36

[35] And when the men of that place had knowledge of him, they sent out into all that country round about, and brought unto him all that were diseased; [36] And besought him that they might only touch the hem of his garment: and as many as touched were made perfectly whole.

Although these people were in the presence of the power of God's Spirit, they did not request a specific healing but were made perfectly whole. They all touched God.

Matthew 9:20–22

²⁰ And, behold, a woman, which was diseased with an issue of blood twelve years, came behind *him*, and touched the hem of his garment: ²¹ For she said within herself, If I may but touch his garment, I shall be whole. ²² But Jesus turned him about, and when he saw her, he said, Daughter, be of good comfort; thy faith hath made thee whole. And the woman was made whole from that hour.

In this miracle there was no verbal request for a specific healing; however, since, in the close presence of the Lord's power all disease is healed, she had only to touch Him. The command to be healed in Hebrews 12:13 is coupled with the Lord's expressing distaste for the fruit of sin—not necessarily performed by the sufferer but perhaps from previous generations, as in genetic diseases. Sin is the foundation for all illness, disease, and deformity—including genetic problems (so-called since genetic changes actually result from other causes and are not the root problem). God always commanded that the sacrifices of the Israelites be without blemish. This seeming demand for perfection in Hebrews 12:13 concerned Bruce, since he still had obvious joint deformities, until he read the following:

Luke 14:21

²¹ So that servant came, and shewed his lord these things. Then the master of the house being angry said to his servant, Go out quickly into the streets and lanes of the city, and bring in hither the poor, and the maimed, and the halt, and the blind.

Healing is likely when our spirit is in the presence of God.

There is a strong principle tying the closeness of a person to the presence of God and the completeness of the application of Psalm 103:1-5 in his life. The question then is how we can learn to be led by the Spirit of God and mortify the flesh. This, learning to have a continually thankful heart, and perfecting continual praise are going to be a great blessing to God. God is blessed when:

1. we truly and completely fulfill the first commandment;

2. one has a meek and contrite spirit;

3. one praises God continually by his lips for the things God is doing in his life;

4. one obeys and honors his parents;

5. one obeys all of the commandments; and

6. one does all of God's work well.

7. in addition, the person:

    a. must mature in his spirit;

    b. must be obedient always to God's commandments in taking his thoughts captive (2 Corinthians 10:5);

    c. must renew the spirit of his mind (Ephesians 4:23); and

    d. must purify his heart (1 Timothy 1:5 and 2 Timothy 2:22).

    e. *These above four commandments are completely overlooked by the Church and by most people; and yet they form the very basis for anything that we can offer to God with which He will be pleased with and which might bless Him.*

To obey God, we must be led by His Spirit.

Obedience to God's commandments (not just an occasional one, but all of them) is part of the basis for how He measures our love for Him.

John 14:15

¹⁵ If ye love me, keep my commandments.

Being Led by the Spirit of God

Our first book *How to be Led by the Spirit of God: Maturing in the Spirit* gives a lot of the Scriptural basis that is important to understand and to keep in memory, in order to learn how to be led by God's Spirit. Our book *Spirit* adds more specific detail and some diagrams based on the content of the first book. We have greater understanding of God's desires for men since writing these books. In them we emphasized the need to take one's thoughts captive, to renew the spirit of his mind, and to develop a pure heart. At this point we add that we should develop a heart that overflows with thankfulness to God and offers a continual sacrifice of praise. In Chapter 3 we gave a brief review of the pathways which we established in our first two books for renewing the mind and purifying the heart. We will now add the need of continual thanksgiving, of continual praise, and of being a blessing to God in order to draw on God's mercy for healing.

When one draws near to God He will draw near to that person. We have to make the first move, but the Spirit of God does quicken our interest in doing that. It all moves toward fulfilling the first commandment. Sadly, few if any people in the Western world come anywhere near fulfilling it. The command to love God includes developing a strong emotional component to the actions, beliefs, and attitudes which demonstrate love. It demands that we always place God's interests, needs, and desires ahead of our own.

Later in this chapter we will add further detail to what we wrote in Chapter 3 about being led by the Spirit of God.

James 4:8

[8] Draw nigh to God, and he will draw nigh to you. Cleanse *your* hands, *ye* sinners; and purify *your* hearts, *ye* double minded.

God uses illness to get a person's attention.

God uses illness to get the attention of people to make changes in their lives. This is why the command to be healed given in Hebrews 12:13 is accompanied by the discussion of punishment for sin. Just a few of the other Scriptures that link sin and illness appear below. The sin might have been from an ancestor and may follow family members as a familial evil cursing spirit. Such spirits need to have their hold broken. This hold is broken at the second birth because a person is now in a new family; and old ties no longer hold. This should be declared. These familial spirits frequently will try to reattach themselves, ignoring the new legal rights the person has after his second birth. However, as one resists any spirit, it will eventually flee from him.

Matthew 9:6

[6] But that ye may know that the Son of man hath power on earth to forgive sins, (then saith he to the sick of the palsy,) Arise, take up thy bed, and go unto thine house.

James 5:16

[16] Confess *your* faults one to another, and pray one for another, that ye may be healed. The effectual fervent prayer of a righteous man availeth much.

Psalm 25:18

[18] Look upon mine affliction and my pain; and forgive all my sins.

The causes of illness

The devil and disease are large topics, and we are going to deal with them in Chapter 7. Sin in the Garden of Eden introduced all illness, infirmity, and death in the flesh for the whole of mankind (Romans 5:12).

God at times will burden people with a specific illness to get their attention. There are many examples in the Scriptures, including Miriam (Moses' sister) being given leprosy for speaking against Moses.

Numbers 12:10

¹⁰ And the cloud departed from off the tabernacle; and, behold, Miriam *became* leprous, *white* as snow: and Aaron looked upon Miriam, and, behold, *she was* leprous.

While it was not for sin, Lazarus was allowed to die so that the Lord Jesus Christ could glorify His Father in raising Lazarus from death after four days had passed.

There are many other examples of God's using physical illness and infirmity for His various purposes.

Exodus 15:26

²⁶ And said, If thou wilt diligently hearken to the voice of the LORD thy God, and wilt do that which is right in his sight, and wilt give ear to his commandments, and keep all his statutes, I will put none of these diseases upon thee, which I have brought upon the Egyptians: for I *am* the LORD that healeth thee.

This Scripture from Exodus shows a very direct link between not listening to God speaking to one as an individual and being prone to illnesses. We feel that this specific issue is a major reason that many children of God are not being healed of physical complaints. In this situation there is spiritual deafness which needs to be healed also. There is almost always a spiritual disease associated with a physical illness. People need to seek healing for both if they are to have a good chance of maintaining a physical healing given to them by God. Healing of spiritual issues will come with maturing in the spirit as one learns to be led by the Spirit of God.

Maturing in the inner man (spirit)

It would be easy to learn how to do this if we did not have two separate forces trying to prevent our being easily led by the Spirit of God. These are the demonic powers and the flesh. The flesh is at least as big a disturbance as the evil spirits are. We listed above the commands in Scripture which help to bring maturity and which must be obeyed. We again emphasize that these are not optional; they are the only way to learn how to be led by the Spirit of God. Being led by the Spirit of God is an essential step in the process of maturing in one's inner man.

One most important point is that God speaks to us frequently through the Scriptures by either bringing a passage to our attention as we are reading it or recalling it to our mind. To the extent that we do not have a good knowledge of the Scriptures we are deaf and blind to the Spirit of God. One cannot walk after the Spirit of God without developing a growing knowledge of the Scriptures—by diligently meditating on them in depth and studying them along topic lines. A daily exposure for 30 to 60 minutes is a bare minimum. We are well aware that few people do this. A passive or cursory reading will not work. One has to be talking with and interacting with the Holy Spirt, who is appointed to lead each of us into all truth. About the only other reference needed is a printed or an electronic concordance. For many reasons the New King James Version is probably the easiest translation that is reasonably accurate for most people to; but it is not as error free as the original Authorized King James version. Many more recent translations have significant errors. The Holy Spirit will help one understand the older English used in the King James Version.

This lack of seriousness with God by many in the faith is a very grave issue for the Church of the Lord (His Body). One can never learn to be led consistently by the Spirit of God without this very serious approach to studying the Bible. At the best, people will then be like the carnal Christians in the Corinthian Church; and while God is merciful and kind, He will likely not let such people have the deeper blessings that He can provide.

One needs to have Scripture knowledge to discern the origin of the thoughts and the origin of the emotions coming into his mind. Evil spirits are great mimics and will misquote Scripture in order to deceive.

A second point is the profound principle in Scripture underlying the taking of thoughts captive. One has to start with small steps in learning to be led by the Spirit of God. Without beginning at the basics, one can never lay a good foundation. People with intellectual gifting sometimes stumble at this, since they might try to use their gift to short-circuit the needed training. The Scriptures tell us that we need to be faithful in the least things, or we cannot be faithful in the larger things. The Lord makes this statement, and He knows how He designed and built our minds and our character. We must trust Him, believe this, and take the small steps. The Scripture below explains this principle.

Luke 16:10

[10] He that is faithful in that which is least is faithful also in much: and he that is unjust in the least is unjust also in much.

A third point to mention is that before one starts the process of maturing he will not really be able to discern his own spirit as a separate entity to his mind or his soul. As one matures, he will become gradually more aware of his inner man.

A fourth point to mention is that the flesh after the second birth still has its old ideas, un-renewed mind, old motivations, actual physical body, and old life goals. It is actually an independent person. Since the Scriptures tell us that the flesh is always at enmity with the Spirit of God and since our new spirit given at the second birth is of God and from God, the flesh also permanently remains antagonistic to the new inner man. This flesh can be very deceptive; it can be subtle; and it will not act in the best interests of a soul after the second birth. After the second birth a soul's best interests are served by following his inner man as the Holy Spirit leads him. The flesh was judged as evil by God, and it is. One should get the image firmly in mind that he really is two people— an inner man and a flesh man (the old man after the second birth). The two are always opposed, and God commands us to "put on" the new man. See the Scriptures below. The new man is the combination of the new spirit and the soul as it is led by the new spirit. It has to be put on (Ephesians 4:24, below).

Romans 8:7

[7] Because the carnal mind [old mind of the flesh] *is* enmity against God: for it is not subject to the law of God, neither indeed can be.

Galatians 5:17

[17] For the flesh lusteth against the Spirit, and the Spirit against the flesh: and these are contrary the one to the other: so that ye cannot do the things that ye would.

Ephesians 4:24

[24] And that ye put on the new man, which after God is created in righteousness and true holiness.

Ephesians 4:23

[23] And be renewed in the spirit of your mind.

A fifth point is that we (soul) have a mind which is independent of the mind of our spirit and also independent of the mind of the flesh. It is our highest-level mind and our highest-level decision making mind. It is this mind that we have to use to sort out the origin of the thoughts coming into it which suggest speech and actions that we can take. These thoughts come from one of several places, but in most cases they will come to the mind of the soul from the heart, as we discussed in Chapter 3.

Some more detail to supplement that in Chapters 3 and 4 about being led by the Spirit of God

The steps of renewing the spirit of the mind, taking thoughts captive, and purifying the heart are all designed by God to help a person communicate with Him more surely and to help him mature in his new abode in the spiritual realm. If a person continually goes through of these three processes, he will eventually fulfill Hebrews 4:12 successfully (which we will discuss below). One's commitment and effort will determine the overall knowledge of Scripture that he learns from the Holy Spirit and His appointed teachers. A significant lack of Scripture knowledge will limit the fulfillment of Hebrews 4:12.

Hebrews 4:12

[12] For the word of God *is* quick, and powerful, and sharper than any twoedged sword, piercing even to the dividing asunder of soul and spirit, and of the joints and marrow, and *is* a discerner of the thoughts and intents of the heart.

By continuing to go through these three processes, one arrives at a level where he can reasonably reliably know the origin of his thoughts. This is important. When he knows which thoughts come from his new spirit and obeys only these, then he will be led by the Spirit of God.

The four areas mentioned in this Scripture are:

1. The soul

2. The spirit (bearing witness to the Holy Spirit in our heart)

3. The flesh (joints and marrow)

4. The heart—the Word of God discerns the truth of the

thoughts and intents (motivations) of the heart. It helps one to discern the origin of each thought prior to it coming into the heart—whether it originated from the flesh, the spirit, an evil spirit, or the soul. It also helps to discern those thoughts arising in the heart and promoted by one of these same four sources.

Romans 8:16

[16] The Spirit itself beareth witness with our spirit, that we are the children of God.

Amplification of where thoughts may originate include:

1. Our own mind of the soul

2. From the mind of the flesh *via* the heart

3. From the Holy Spirit *via* the inner man and usually *via* the heart

4. From the heart, which is also the place that our imaginations arise

5. From evil spirits that are able to influence in many ways

    a. through the lusts of the flesh *via* the heart or directly to the mind of the soul

    b. through appealing to our vision that sets up lusts and desires for appealing items

    c. through the pride that we have in who we are (pride of life)

    d. through bringing various emotional forces against the soul and planting thoughts into the mind of the soul

God knows all of our thoughts; and in the spiritual realm there is no deceit. The demonic spirits do have ability to know much about our thoughts (not as much as God does), and they have the ability to try to influence them by planting suggestions into the minds of our soul, our heart, and our flesh. This is an ongoing process for those attempting to mature in the spirit. The demonic forces have a numerical advantage in that not many people are even aware that God commands us to mature in our inner man. The demonic forces can closely watch those who are trying to mature; they to make life bothersome for them. None of this attempted influencing of one's thoughts is demonic possession or anything like it.

Neither the old man nor the natural realm man will have any understanding of how he is influenced by demonic thoughts; since neither believes nor has any operating understanding of these issues. These implanted thoughts always try to appeal to a subtle fear—sometimes a not so subtle fear. They atempt to intimidate by fears. Examples of such fears are not performing well at work, losing a job, having insufficient money, and many similar things. These thoughts are just like any of our other thoughts, although there will frequently be pressure along with a persistent and noisy quality. At times these spirits will almost be "in one's face," as it were.

6. God Himself will place thoughts into our spirit, and He will also speak through our external circumstances (see 1 Thessalonians 5:18 should be studied and clearly understood). God has the ability to order all of the events in our lives based on the direction we choose to go, either to Him or away from Him. He orders these events to train us for eternity, which is a major purpose in this natural realm.

7. God sometimes will send angels to speak directly to us. We may not be aware that an angel has addressed us (Hebrews 13:2).

Let us summarize what we have covered.

If we have continued the two cycles of purifying the heart and renewing the mind (we should never stop), then we will have learned how to be in a position of obeying God. We would be nowhere near spiritual maturity at this point, but we would have the tools to start growing in spiritual strength and acquiring spiritual-realm wisdom, understanding, and knowledge. At this point we should become more aware of our self-will.

The self- will is in the old man, and Scripture requires that we put on the new man

Ephesians 4:24

[24] And that ye put on the new man, which after God is created in righteousness and true holiness.

Colossians 3:10

[10] And have put on the new *man*, which is renewed in knowledge after the image of him that created him:

The process of putting on the new man is the daily mortification of the flesh.

Romans 8:13

[13] For if ye live after the flesh, ye shall die: but if ye through the Spirit do mortify the deeds of the body, ye shall live.

The Self-Will

The self-will of the old man is incredibly strong, and it is quite a process to defeat it. Whenever it leads our behavior, we are being led by the flesh; and the actions we take will not be approved by God. Isaiah 64:6 (above) discusses this.

The problem when we work from our flesh (old man) is that God's ways are above ours; His thoughts are higher than ours; and so the initiation of any work (supposedly done for Him) might actually have a negative impact on His plans. In addition, He has also condemned the flesh in all forms. Romans 7:18 speaks about God's view of all fleshly-led acts and statements.

[18] For I know that in me (that is, in my flesh,) dwelleth no good thing: for to will is present with me; but *how* to perform that which is good I find not.

Prior to going through the second birth, we all relied on our self-determinations. We chose what we wished to do, influenced by demonic thoughts unwittingly mingled with our own. Growing up in the world system values, one really had no choice but to help himself. It is very hard to change from this, since we still have an unrenewed mind after the second birth; and we have little understanding at that time of how we can trust God to take care of us. Nonetheless, these acts of our flesh in self-determination will, if not mortified with the rest of our flesh, cause us to have few works to offer God; and the rest will be burned (2 Peter 3:10).

God's Works

God's works for us in this age include the ministry of reconciliation of lost souls to God, the taking back of the works of the devil, and the training of our spirit for the ages to come. God positions His children in all areas of secular work in order for them to be able to influence those with whom they are in contact throughout all societies.

Destroying self-will

Until self-will is destroyed, one will not be able to serve God adequately as a bondservant, a servant, a friend, or in any other capacity.

We noted that when one fulfills Hebrews 4:12, he can tell the source of his thoughts. As he has been learning to do this through the renewal of the mind, he has also been strengthening his spirit; and he has been mortifying his flesh so he is already part of the way to mortifying the self (self-will). As he sets his face to follow only the direction and leading of his spirit, as witnessed to by the Holy Spirit, he will find that his faith in God will grow because he will see how God takes care of him, talks with him, teaches him, loves him, and meets all of his needs. This process allows purification of the heart, as he gives up old things and allows God to build new structures in the heart. All of this helps in destroying the self.

God is the only one who can really help us break the self-will. He does this by leading us into situations which we are not going to find very comfortable. They have to be faced for God to break his will. The Scripture 1 Peter 4:1-2 (below) indicates the process. One might well find the Lord leading him through the Valley of the Shadow of Death (Psalm 23). When one is doing the will of God, he is not following his own will of the flesh. The Lord will present challenges to test his resolve to follow Him until he himself can see that he has developed a much stronger relationship with Him. One has to have a deep relationship with Him through experiences and conversations in order to see that he can trust Him in all areas of his life. One does not want to have a shallow root system which will wither (Luke 8:13) in the testing.

1 Peter 4:1–2

[1] Forasmuch then as Christ hath suffered for us in the flesh, arm yourselves likewise with the same mind: for he that hath suffered in the flesh hath ceased from sin; [2] That he no longer should live the rest of *his* time in the flesh to the lusts of men, but to the will of God.

Suggestions for assisting the Lord God to break the self-will:

1. Meditate on the character and the abilities of God. This need is why we have so much of this book devoted to these aspects of God.

2. Meditate on God's Word frequently.

3. Become strong in the spirit, since this will weaken the flesh.

4. Continue to renew the mind and purify the heart.

5. Contemplate the reality of how much control one really has over his future, and start to see how little skill one has in understanding the spiritual realm without God's teaching you.

6. Set eternity in your heart as you renew your mind.

7. Meditate and reflect on the things God does for you each day and also on the past milestones in your relationship with God.

We have to learn the character of God through our experiences with Him. As we do this, our heart becomes more purified. We have to learn that in the spiritual realm we are totally dependent on our Father for our survival, even for 30 seconds or less. The evil powers would devour us, were it not for our Father's protecting us.

It becomes easier as to resist the devil, stand against him, and ultimately to overcome him (although few accomplish this overcoming) as we work with our Father to be trained in the warfare within the spiritual realm. We can learn how we can use God's Word as a sword against the spiritual powers (Ephesians 6:10-17).

We have to transfer our reliance on the self-developed skills in the natural realm, where we feel independent, to a reliance on the skills of God to protect us and to train us in the spiritual realm.

Gradually, as we experience more of God, know Him better, and draw closer to Him, we will see the issues in the spiritual realm more clearly as God develops our sense of spiritual vision in our inner man. We will find that our requirement for self-importance and self at the center diminishes rapidly as God's all-consuming love embraces us. We can trust Him to care for us in all aspects of our life (Philippians 4:19). The transition to the destruction of the self-will comes from seeing how small we are and how large God is. We will see that we cannot trust ourselves but, we can trust God. All of this comes as we are obedient to do His commands in all aspects.

What is meant by maturing in the spirit (inner man)

When we receive our new spirit from God at the time of the second birth, it comes with an ability to communicate with God the Holy Spirit in a sophisticated and highly intelligent manner. It comes from God and is of God. It resides in the new spiritual heart with no pre-existing structures to interfere with communication from God to the mind of the soul. In God's wisdom at the second birth He leaves the soul with a mind which is to be renewed and which is to transition from a primary and intense focus on the natural realm to a primary and intense focus on the spiritual realm. If the soul chooses to renew the mind, then the soul will be able to walk after the Spirit of God. It will do this by learning to listen to the inner man and to watch what the inner man is seeing and hearing. If the soul fails to make this transition to be focused on watching and listening to the inner man, then by default it will listen to the flesh (and evil spirits speaking through the flesh). The mind has to be renewed in the overall thrust and direction of the thought processes and thought content, It must no longer focus primarily on natural-realm facts and ways of doing things and instead must learn how the spiritual-realm functions and must reason using spiritual-realm truth.

Very few people who have been through the second birth have been instructed in this need to transition from a natural-realm focus to a spiritual-realm focus. Consequently, most people continue to be led by the flesh, although they occasionally listen to and follow the inner man. This results in a carnal Christian walk which the apostle Paul identified as being in the believers in Corinth. When a person fails to renew his mind and continues to be led by the flesh after the second birth, the new heart is quickly made impure; and old structures, motivations, beliefs, and attitudes return to build structures which are opposed to and which block the Spirit of God from flowing through this individual and into the community around him.

The flesh is always at enmity with God and is evil. We have to learn to see this current creation as God sees it—evil, transient, and under judgment. The soul with the new inner man is no longer under God's judgment regarding its eternal destination, but it is still going to be judged on what choices the soul makes regarding being led by the Spirit of God. This judgment results in some of our works being burned and some standing. What we need to do is to understand how our soul can cooperate with God to renew the mind, purify the heart, and thus to be led by the Spirit of God.

Yet another look at how we can renew the mind and purify the heart

The issue of reaching the fulfillment of Hebrews 4:12 is so important that we are going to look at it again with some different thoughts. When the soul allows the flesh to dominate the use of its mind, due to the lack of renewal of it, then the strength of the inner man decreases. The impact of the inner man on the soul and its decision making is small. Conversely, the strength of the inner man increases and that of the flesh decreases when the soul renews the mind to focus on the issues of God and to follow the advice and promptings of the inner man. We read before that the flesh and the spirit are constantly opposed and that the flesh is always opposed to God. Any thoughts, emotions and energy from the flesh is evil in the sight of God, and one must believe that in his spiritual heart. These concepts are going to be quite unusual for many; a person may be somewhat uneasy about them, but that is an area where he has to decide that he believes the Word of God.

The rewards of being led by the Spirit are enormous, but it is always a battle to overcome the influence of the flesh and to go through the rigorous changes in one's goals, motivations, attitudes, and beliefs that are needed to place God first. One must set one's whole energy on learning how to love Him and to bless Him, as the First Commandment requires. We will again review God's formula for making these changes in one's life. We must be very careful to be faithful in the multiple small steps, or we will never be able to be faithful in much. When Scripture states a fact like that in Luke 16:10, God has made man in such a way that it will always be true, regardless of man's ideas about it.

Maturing in the Inner Man (and Soul)

The following list of actions is needed to place a person on the path to maturing in the soul through development and maturing of the inner man. We will deal with them sequentially.

1. Renewing the Mind

2. Purifying the Spiritual Heart

3. Perfecting Worship and Praise

4. Learning to Love the Lord God

5. Blessing the Lord God

6. Restoring the broken relationship between man and God

As one progresses through these steps, his spirit strengthens; and his flesh recedes (Galatians 5:16-17). His spirit also matures in true wisdom, true understanding, and true knowledge.

Renewing the Mind

Romans 12:2 commands us to renew our minds.

2 And be not conformed to this world: but be ye transformed by the renewing of your mind, that ye may prove what is that good, and acceptable, and perfect, will of God.

The *path* to renewing the mind is based on the following command of God:

2 Corinthians 10:5

⁵ Casting down imaginations, and every high thing that exalteth itself against the knowledge of God, and bringing into captivity every thought to the obedience of Christ.

These imaginations and high things are beliefs, attitudes, motivations, and goals in the heart, which are incompatible in some areas with the truth in the Scripture. These have to be torn down with God's help, and new structures which He alone can build must be erected. He will build the right fortresses, refuges, and strong towers in the "city" of the heart.

The Scripture commands us to bring every thought, planned act, motivation, goal, belief, and attitude into a consistency with Scripture and which, when performed well, will leave the individual with a servant like dependency on God. All of one's energy will come from the Spirit of God, as a branch is attached to a vine. This is like living within the envelope of God's character and mind, thus making Him our habitation (Psalm 91:9). We have to end up with the same beliefs, attitudes, decisions, character, and actions that God Himself has. We have to have the Lord Jesus Christ formed in our heart.

Galatians 4:19

¹⁹ My little children, of whom I travail in birth again until Christ be formed in you,

This does not happen overnight. It is only completed successfully as one does this taking of thoughts captive consistently, thought by thought. He must reject those thoughts which do not measure up to Scripture as taught by the Holy Spirit. He should not put into speech or action anything that is not pleasing to God, and he has to wait for God to speak to him personally about any significant changes in his life to see what God wishes for him. He should look at each thought to see what the motive behind it is. If it is elevating self, reject it; if it is elevating God, perform it. He should speak to God and listen constantly. He must keep his heart joyful and at peace all the time in order to improve his ability to communicate with God. Restlessness and anxiety tend to make it hard to discern the origin of our thoughts, except we know that any fear and anxiety will not be from the Spirit of God. However, the evil powers attack the thoughts from God and try to prevent our acting on them. This secondary attack is designed to paralyze actions. Whenever our inner peace and joy are not present, this alerts us to an attack on the inner man from the flesh or from an evil spirit; it requires action to identify the threat and block it. Frequently, we will need to ask God to give us power over the spirit causing the loss of peace and joy. The two scriptures below address this.

Romans 14:17

[17] For the kingdom of God is not meat and drink; but righteousness, and peace, and joy in the Holy Ghost.

Ephesians 3:16

[16] That he would grant you, according to the riches of his glory, to be strengthened with might by his Spirit in the inner man;

In Chapter 5 we discussed how even a simple decision to run an errand has to be examined for timing (is it really needed, or is it a way of filling in time)? It may just simply be to serve a family need.

It is obvious that the more Scripture one knows the better able he will be to take thoughts captive properly. Renewing the mind is a continuous process, and at times it can be quite a difficult process. Only God can effectively teach it. It must be done to lay a firm foundation for further development. Initially, one has to be renewed in the spirit of the mind. This means turning from self will, and thinking in the natural realm to become focused on the spiritual realm and to seek God's will. At first, it might feel awkward; but after several weeks or months it will become more automatic. At the same time one is doing this, he should be intensively studying Scripture from a good translation. We highly recommend, for several reasons, the New King James or the King James version, as being most accurate in core doctrine with the original languages. As this process goes on, then one gradually brings His mind captive to the mind of the Lord Jesus Christ.

Keep an overall perspective about taking thoughts captive.

At the outset one should keep in mind some overall guides. He must understand that He is trying to let God develop the senses of his inner man—touch, taste, smell, position sense, and (most of all) hearing and seeing. As one goes through the above cycle of taking thoughts captive, studying Scripture, and then making further adjustments to his attitudes, motivations, and beliefs, he is renewing the spirit of his mind. The renewal should have the goals of communicating better with God and of being trained to operate in the spiritual realm as far as God needs him to during this phase of his life. One's spirit is seated with God in the heavens (Ephesians 2:6), even as it dwells in his flesh. Renewing the spirit of the mind should include developing the love for God commanded in the First Commandment. One should be very cautious about anything that does not seem to fit these overall goals.

We must greatly question everything that we learned under the world system prior to the second birth as most of it is at the foundation false wisdom, false understanding, and false knowledge. We must seek that true wisdom, true understanding, and true knowledge which come from the spiritual realm and which explain the natural realm laws of mechanics as a stability provided by God for constancy, understanding that these are not universal laws and are frequently overruled by the miraculous. God's working of miracles is designed to change relationships between Him and people. One needs to understand that many spiritual realm laws are based on relationships between individual spirit beings, such as a man's having faith in God. There are spiritual-realm laws regarding spiritual matter, but God has not revealed much about these in the Scriptures. We know that God directly supplies all of the power for this regulation of spiritual matter, although He delegates some to his angelic hosts. In addition, God delegates a small amount of this specific use of power to man.

The separation of flesh, heart, spirit, and soul is the overall goal of taking thoughts captive.

We discussed this separation before (Hebrews 4:12 above). Another look will be helpful. One can learn to understand the components of all spiritual communications (power, emotion, and information) and use them as a means of identifying what planned speech and behavior to allow and which to block in order to strengthen the spirit over the flesh. Over time the flesh will be weakened; the inner man will be strengthened; one will become much more aware of his inner man; and one can be led by the Spirit of God. One will be able to identify accurately thoughts from God (*via* the inner man), from the flesh, from the heart, and from the soul. One will see that this fulfills the Scripture of Hebrews 4:12.

Strengthening the spirit

Each decision we make to follow our inner man is really following God's direction, since the Holy Spirit informs our inner man of His purposes for us. Performing God's directives strengthens our spirit, even in common daily repetitive decisions. We must mortify the flesh in all that we say and do. The flesh does not profit us in eternity.

Romans 8:13

[13] For if ye live after the flesh, ye shall die: but if ye through the Spirit do mortify the deeds of the body, ye shall live.

Hebrews 4:12

[12] For the word of God *is* quick [alive], and powerful, and sharper than any twoedged sword, piercing even to the dividing asunder of soul and spirit, and of the joints and marrow, and *is* a discerner of the thoughts and intents of the heart.

The ability to identify the source of a thought is the major goal when taking thoughts captive. There is a heavy dependency on the Scripture in performing this discernment. It is the knowledge of the Scripture interpreted by the Holy Spirit, as opposed to the tradition of men, which is the foundation for this separation. When one can reliably do this identification, then he can be led by the Spirit of God, if he will act in belief on those thoughts from God.

The renewal of the mind must be accompanied by purifying the heart. We will look at how this is accomplished briefly and will address it in more detail in Chapter 7.

Purifying the Spiritual Heart

Acts 15:9 commands the purifying of the heart.

Acts 15:9

[9] And put no difference between us and them, purifying their hearts by faith.

This purification is a process of removing those evil strongholds and imaginations in the fleshly dominated heart. It involves changing evil beliefs, attitudes, goals, and motivations (evil is anything built as a defense against coming to the knowledge of God). It is done through faith. As we hear God make a statement to us individually or through the Scripture (as a word that the Holy Spirit highlights to us), then we act in belief on this; and over time God is able to tear down old structures in our heart and build new ones. As we take thoughts captive, we need to see if it is from God, or the flesh, or the heart, or even an evil spirit. This process is a spiritual battle. We have to grasp the fact that God designed man with the potential to fight an internal war, which is the inner man versus what we have to view as a potentially mortal enemy, the flesh.

When we act in belief on the thoughts from God His advice to us, then we start to trust Him over time, as we see that His advice is always for our good. It can take a lot of standing strong, as evil spirits and the flesh cry out and send multitudes of opposing thoughts to our mind. Evil spirits and the flesh will try intimidation to block us from acting on a word from God; and they may be quite persistent before they will flee from us (James 4:7) in conformance to the Word of God. These processes are not always easy, but this is what it takes if one is to develop a pure heart. A pure heart will seek the company of God above working for Him; it will seek to be in His presence where there is fullness of joy and peace forever. God will test us to strengthen us and to show us what is still in need of change. Small things lead to larger things; we should never despise small beginnings. As we trust Him, we start to understand His character; and this leads to the blessings of Psalm 91:14-16.

Perfecting praise and worship

When we praise the Lord individually, it needs to be based on the many things that He has done for us; and it should be based on His character. It can be noisy, with music and with uplifted hands, or standing. The emotions of gratitude and of thanksgiving should accompany it. It should not be done as a rote performance. Praise can also be done in a corporate worship setting to which one would go, again in gratitude for the things the Lord has done for him.

Praise should be free-flowing and not with any vain repetition. When one looks at all of the things which occur during a day and does this to see what God is doing in each circumstance to further the eternal future for an himself, then he should be able to praise easily. He can also praise God by recounting major things that He has done in his life.

Perfected praise brings one into the courts of the Lord (into His presence). One should continue to praise until he senses the peace and joy of being in the presence of God. At this point he will be able to praise as the Spirit of God directs.

Worship is an adoration of the Lord for all He is to a person. Again there is the need to worship the Lord for personal kindness and grace He has given to one. Worship is to be done in the beauty of holiness (Psalm 29:2). One can worship the Lord in a manner pleasing to Him only if he keeps his life separated from the world system. The world system should have no emotional hold on him. He should have no affection for the flesh, since the Lord states that the flwsh is of no useful purpose unless it is subject in all things to a strong inner man. We must view the flesh in the same way as the Lord does and not be distracted by it. We must be anxious for nothing; for all anxiety is rooted in the flesh.

To worship the Lord, we have to know Him well. Obviously, as we has more years after the second birth, our praise and worship should be richer in experience and deeper in personal knowledge of the Lord God. If it is not, then repentance is required; and we need to make a new beginning under God's direction. We need to thank Him for His salvation, for His creation, for our future with Him, for the power He gives us, for the healing that He gives us, and many more things. When one is not holy, worship is not going to be received as well, since it will be mixed with fleshly thinking. We have to have our focus on eternity, being with Him, and being His child.

John 6:63

[63] It is the spirit that quickeneth; the flesh profiteth nothing: the words that I speak unto you, *they* are spirit, and *they* are life.

Psalm 29:2

[2] Give unto the LORD the glory due unto his name; worship the LORD in the beauty of holiness.

In the next chapter we will paint a deeper and broader understanding of the flesh and the wicked designs it has for us. It is probably the greatest enemy of the soul. The flesh would like to see us at enmity with God for eternity. We have to strengthen our inner man (this results in weakening the flesh) in order to be able to praise and worship God adequately.

Enhancing praise and worship of God through strengthening the inner man

God commands us to worship Him in spirit and in truth. Thus, any strengthening of our inner man will lead to enhanced ability to praise and worship Him. Some ways to strengthen our spirit are to praise and worship God several times a day; to seek God to strengthen us in the inner man (Ephesians 3:16); to focus on maturing in the spirit which comes as one renews the mind and purifies the heart; and to set our hearts on eternity (which orders our priorities).

Perhaps the most important way to strengthen our spirit is to pray in the spirit using our prayer language (praying in the Holy Spirit [Jude 20]). This is very important for strengthening the inner man since he will be using our flesh to speak to the Lord God. This action subjects the flesh very directly. The flesh will try to ridicule our attempts to use our prayer language. We must say "no" to the flesh always.

Jude 20

[20] But ye, beloved, building up yourselves on your most holy faith, praying in the Holy Ghost.

Jude 21 states another powerful way to strengthen the spirit. One's spirit is always weakened by active fear (active fear means those with which we have not dealt). Since perfect love casts out fear, then keeping in the love of God eliminates the fear.

Jude 21

²¹ Keep yourselves in the love of God, looking for the mercy of our Lord Jesus Christ unto eternal life.

God always loves us, but we do not always receive it; thus, the commands us to keep ourselves in the love of God. When we purify our heart to accept God's love continually, then we are able to have fear cast out of our heart by the love coming into our heart from God. This greatly strengthens our spirit, because love always has a very positive impact on both the one receiving it and the one bestowing it. Fear is always from an evil spirit; and as we are perfected in the perfect love of God, no evil spirit will be able to impact our heart.

1 John 4:18

¹⁸ There is no fear in love; but perfect love casteth out fear: because fear hath torment. He that feareth is not made perfect in love.

Learning to love the Lord God

It is very difficult for a person who has just been through the second birth to come to love the Lord God truly with the emotional accompaniment that is associated with this word *love*.

The flesh is so used to substituting lust for love in people that it is very likely many people will not even know what the emotion of Godly love is really like. We cannot love God with the same weak and impure emotions people would describe as love. God even makes it easy for new spiritual infants. He just demands that they show love through being obedient to the words He speaks directly to them and that He speaks by highlighting a Scripture for a situation they may be facing.

As one gains experiences with the Lord, he learns that it is only as he spends time in God's presence—with the fullness of joy and peace that accompany this—that he begins to develop affection for God. It is in recalling of all of the Lord's interactions with one that he will see the character of the Lord operating in his life. This will increase his gratitude to God and his affection for God.

As the evil of the world system and the destructive impact of the flesh become apparent to a person, then he will also realize that even the desire to do work for God is in need of gradual replacement by a desire just to be in His presence, because of the pleasurable way he feels. After this point he begins to experience love for God as he sees that the Lord really is working out everything for his eternal good, that being in His presence is supportive and enjoyable, and that he is finding a growing concern to see God honored and worshiped. He will also have a concern to see evil vanquished. He will love the character and the works of God.

None of this change in one's love for God happens overnight. It takes a lot of spiritual energy and power to come to love God in an emotionally strong manner, because the flesh resists actively most of the way and is assisted by evil spirits which lend it power.

God runs to help His child when He sees that individual's heart is set on learning to love Him for who He is.

(Luke 15:20

[20] And he arose, and came to his father. But when he was yet a great way off, his father saw him, and had compassion, and ran, and fell on his neck, and kissed him.

Getting to love God involves seeing His character in many situations and seeing His work in one's life over time. Psalm 91:14 describes the benefits God gives to one who knows His character.

Blessing the Lord God

We discussed this topic extensively in Chapter 2.

Retoring the broken relationship with God

If we perform the actions in the five points discussed for maturing in the inner man as a means to improve the likelihood of receiving healing from God, we will have walked a long way on the path described in Scripture for restoring the relationship of man with God, which was broken in the Garden of Eden. Additionally, we must increase our love for and adoration of God above all else.

This broken relationship between God and man is the basis for all illness, disease, and infirmity. Restoring this properly is a great blessing for both God and man. As this relationship is healed, all spiritual and physical illness will be healed in a parallel manner. Only God can determine when a person (or a group of people) is doing this properly. Healings come as the maturing soul gets back into the correct relationship with God, as God is pleased and as God is blessed.

Healing will come (Psalm 103)

Healing will come as the Spirit of God strengthens us and courses through us into the community around us. Healing is such a part of God that it happens when He is present, even for judgment, since judgment brings healing from strife.

Healing comes as one labors in prayer before God to be filled with His peace, joy, and power. God has honored that request in our lives (quickly at times). When God brings His presence into one's heart, then evil spirits and the flesh will give way (1 John 4:18—[printed just above]). Evil spirits are always associated with fear, and perfect love in one's heart will cause them to flee.

We should not confuse this sequence of renewing the mind, purifying the heart, praising, praying, and blessing God as our performing a work to be rewarded with healing. It is faith and belief in the heart that God will fulfill His Words in the Scripture. This faith and belief in the heart increase greatly, as we start to love God, as we experience His love for us, and as we draw close to Him.

We are not loving God if we perform these acts just to be healed.

That would be using Him. It is acceptable to decide that we want the benefits God offers in Psalm 103:1-5; He actually tells us to search out His benefits (in the original language of Psalm 103:2). As we start to learn how to bless God, we are going to be drawn into loving Him, however weakly and incompletely. He is so kind that He will draw niear to us quickly as we draw near to Him.

The Flesh

In the next chapter we will look at the mortal enemies of healing in both the spirit and the flesh. One is the flesh itself, perhaps surprising that it would not want God's healing, but understandable since in the presence of God the flesh is very weak. The other enemies are the evil spirits, which tend to work through the flesh of individuals by accentuating fear in various areas including in the heart and in the mind of the soul.

The Church

The current structure and operations of the church in the West have caused it inadvertently to become a stumbling block for more healing from God to be manifest. While not actually an enemy of God, the Church is weak and is generally of little help for individuals who are seeking divine healing. We will look at some issues that God has given us to ponder regarding this situation in Chapter 8.

The Enemies of Healing

Chapter Seven

We have discussed that we do not see many healings given by God in our churches currently. There is confusion in the minds of many people who have medical treatment and credit God with healing. He is to be credited, in a general sense, with these healings, since it is God who has provided the knowledge for physicians to perform their work.

Healing by God, by contrast, as portrayed in the Scriptures is given supernaturally, and there is no human action other than such things as the laying on of hands and the act of praying to God for His involvement. Healing by God is superior by far to that given by physicians. There are no side effects; there are no surgical scars; and there is restoration of function without additional therapy such as physical therapy, occupational therapy, and other various treatment modalities. There are people raised from death (this still happens in many parts of the world); people are healed spiritually and physically; and sin is forgiven frequently in association with the physical healing.

The Lord Jesus equated sickness with sin many times, as in the Scripture below. The original sin led to the entry into the natural realm of illness and death of the flesh. There is always sin involved with sickness and illness, but sometimes it is in ancestors and not necessarily in the one who is ill. The Lord Jesus Christ equated healing of sin and illness as consistent with the work of a physician (Mark 2:16-17). In a real sense he was titling Himself as a physician. One can safely state that spiritual illness and physical illness result from sin. Both need to be healed at the same time; if the spiritual illness is not addressed, the physical healing might not survive a demonic attack. James 5:14-16 indicates that sin has to be forgiven or confessed for the healing to occur.

God commands His children to be healed by Him (Hebrews 12:13); and when this does not happen, one should seek an explanation and correct sin issues made by himself so that he can be healed. Many people think that the story in Mark 7:24-30 shows that the prayer request to be given our daily bread is consistent with a request for healing; when prayed daily one could be requesting good health. Early in Chapter 6 we listed reasons that God's children develop illness and infirmity. Many of these involve situations which require action from the individual in order for God to heal him. There is no guarantee in Scripture that God will heal those who are not His children; but He is gracious, kind, and merciful. In addition, He has healed many people who did not come into a relationship with Him. Since He does not change in His character, it is very likely that a person coming before Him to petition for healing would receive, it provided that he comes to the God who authored the Scriptures.

Mark 2:16–17

[16] And when the scribes and Pharisees saw him eat with publicans and sinners, they said unto his disciples, How is it that he eateth and drinketh with publicans and sinners? [17] When Jesus heard *it*, he saith unto them, They that are whole have no need of the physician, but they that are sick: I came not to call the righteous, but sinners to repentance.

Faith and healing

One must never presume on God when he does not have the faith to believe God for healing. This is a sin of presumption, and this sin can lead to discipline from God. The early churches needed correction of several errors. One was about what is lawful in terms of eating and abstaining from various foods, and another concerned which days one should worship. The apostle Paul described these issues as involving spiritual maturity and the correct state of the conscience (Romans 14). He found no laws regarding these issues but considered them issues of conscience and described a need not to offend a person with a weaker conscience.

God does not seem to regard going to a physician as sin for most people, but it is not going to give the best healing. There is no condemnation of any who go to physicians in the Scriptures other than King Asa. Luke was not condemned for his work as a physician. However, for those in leadership (King Asa) there was condemnation for not requesting healing from God instead of going to a physician. Going to a physician or not going to a physician depends on what level of faith and belief one has, and one must humbly accept this. Pride could easily lead one to "dig his heels in" for approval of men and say he is waiting on God for healing. We should always ask God what He wants us to do in each situation. The answer may well vary from illness to illness.

2 Chronicles 16:12

[12] And Asa in the thirty and ninth year of his reign was diseased in his feet, until his disease *was* exceeding *great*: yet in his disease he sought not to the LORD, but to the physicians.

With the obvious superiority and power in healings given by God the question arises as to why one would not seek this option automatically over the other options of going to a physician or other health-care providers. The answer is that the activity of the flesh and the activity of evil spirits cause confusion of the minds and hardening the hearts of those seeking healing. Hardening of the heart blunts the spiritual senses of vision and hearing. In the Church in the West many people have hard hearts. They may even see miracles in other people, but their heart and mind do not deal with the information due to the hardness in the heart. Without reasoning they will seek just a natural realm solution for their health concerns. We, also, have been guilty of this. However, we, your authors, have both been given healing directly by God; and we can attest to the truth of our statements. Moreover, we have both seen people healed form terminal disease; and we have heard first-hand accounts from pastors we knew very well who have seen people raised from death. Getting rid of hardness of the heart is something which requires much spiritual energy and work.

We shall explore the issues of the flesh and its role in causing hardness of the heart; and we will explore how demons cause difficulty with healing by confusing individuals and by casting a spirit of confusion, doubt, and lack of faith over wide geographic areas. Before we look at the role the flesh plays and the way demons interact with people, we need to take a more detailed look at the spiritual heart.

The Spiritual Heart

Since the spiritual heart is a spiritual structure, it is not surprising that it contains spiritual structures. We have discussed that there are no natural-realm equivalents in terms of the structure of the spiritual heart. This heart is a complex structure, for God sees the structure and content as who we are before Him. Scripture records that the following items are found in the spiritual heart—an intelligent mind; a table(s); idols (these are not necessarily false gods but rather the things on which we spend our time, our resources, and our energy efforts; imaginations; and high places. The Law of God is written in hearts; things can be hidden in them; meditation can be performed in them; evil spirits can dwell in them; mercy and truth can be written on the tables; letters and documents can be written in them; and they contain the Holy Spirit after the second birth. They also contain the inner man. They contain many devices (plans and schemes). The conscience is on the surface of the heart. Hearts vary in size and can be large and deep.

We can look at the heart as containing a spiritual city with various streets, paths, highways, and many buildings. There are walls and barricades. After our birth and until one goes through the second birth the flesh has the most input into the streets and buildings we erect in our hearts. Demonic influence lends input, usually without our noticing it, into what we erect. A desire to protect themselves and/or to promote themselves motivates most people in selecting which structures to build. Sometimes the self is threatened by the thought of having to come into a relationship with God. This is more clearly understood in the spiritual realm. The spirit of man tries to hide from God. The reaction of Adam and Eve after the original sin (Genesis 3:9-10) shows this. Many of the structures we build in the heart are barriers to keep God away. None entirely succeed; and we can see a partial image of God in most people.

We looked before at the fact that the content of one's heart actually has a profound impact on the outward appearance of the flesh of the body. We gave the example of King Nebuchadnezzar. His was an extreme example. Since the content of most hearts is not extremely different from that of other people's hearts, we should not look at the external appearance of an individual to diagnose the content of his spiritual heart. The appearance of the flesh is certainly not an accurate tool for diagosing recent changes, because the flesh will usually change more slowly than the content of the heart. A person with the spiritual gift of discernment and a spiritually mature person will be able to assess partially the content of a spiritual heart.

We have discussed that there is always a link between spiritual illnesses and physical illnesses. There are many abnormal states of the heart mentioned in Scripture—such as anxiety, rebellion, fearfulness, sorrowfulness, impenitence, evil, pain, deceit, perverseness, and heaviness—which indicate a diseased heart. We know even from natural realm observations that disease in the heart impacts the health of the flesh. An example is anxiety with the associated psychosomatic illnesses including high blood pressure, cardiac disease, diabetes, thyroid disease, peptic ulcers, and irritable bowel disease. In order to heal spiritual problems, one needs after going through the second birth to come into a healthy and developing relationship with God. Disease in the spiritual heart results from sin, from poor spiritual food, or from a lack of spiritual food. The Word of God is the right food and provides much spiritual energy for growth and healing in the heart.

The State of the Heart after the Second Birth

At the second birth God gives an individual a new heart. If a person could be trained immediately in how to develop and grow in the spiritual realm and in how to relate directly to God, then the his life might be entirely different. As it is, we have never met such a person. Since people are not given a new mind at the second birth, they quickly have the new heart polluted by many of the same things found in the old heart. The description above is of a heart prior to the second birth. After the second birth there will not be quite the same barriers to God; but whenever the soul makes decisions which allow the flesh to be strong in comparison to the inner man, it will subtly build structures which minimize the input from God and from the spiritual realm. By the time a person realizes this, there will be a lot of work to be done to get the heart into a condition that God desires. Changing the structures and content of the heart involves a lot of spiritual power and energy. Change is never easy because the flesh and evil spirits aiding the flesh pour energy into countering the change. There can be quite an extended war for the control of the heart (flesh versus spirit).

In the heart four structures—faith, hope, belief, and love—that we build are very important and relate to the way the spiritual heart operates in terms of working with God and drawing out His benefits to His children. Love is the most important of these factors, and we will discuss it further with its role in obtaining God's benefits for His children (1 Corinthians 13:13).

Faith, Hope, and Belief in the Heart

Many promises of God are dependent on one having faith in God, and having belief in the spiritual heart (as opposed to the mind of the soul). Mark 11:23-24 is a very broad promise related to those beliefs which we hold in our heart.

How demonic spirits see us

We should note that the demons also know what we hold in our heart. In fact, the demons see us as we see ourselves. An important Scripture which demonstrates this is that of the spies that-Moses sent into the Promised Land. Ten of those who came back related that there were giants in the land. Furthermore, they related how that they saw themselves as grasshoppers and that this caused the giants to do the same. This insight given to the giants came through demonic idea planting. This Scripture is a foundational one for spiritual warfare. It shows that to fight spiritual warfare successfully we have to allow God to change our self image, which is in our heart, to reflect a deep understanding of spiritual-realm truth regarding God, His character, the relative strength of God and demons, and God's protective relationship with His people. The other two spies, Caleb and Joshua, because of their understanding of these spiritual realm truths, came back ready to go into the Promised Land, presuming with faith and belief, that God would overcome the giants.

In addition, God sees us for who we are from our spiritual heart (Proverbs 27:19). To be successful in spiritual warfare, we have to:

1. Strengthen our image of the character of God and of how He will take care of us.

2. See the relative strength of the demonic spirits in comparison to God.

3. Strengthen our relationship with God and let Him build faith and belief in our hearts.

Numbers 13:33

[33] And there we saw the giants, the sons of Anak, *which come* of the giants: and we were in our own sight as grasshoppers, and so we were in their sight.

Defining Hope

Following we have a list of Scriptures which deal with hope and which are representative of how hope is used.

Romans 8:20

²⁰ For the creature was made subject to vanity, not willingly, but by reason of him who hath subjected *the same* in hope.

God subjected the creation to vanity at the time of the fall of man. The creation will be replaced at the end of this age. During this age it has been largely cut off from the life-giving Spirit of God. When God subjected the creation to vanity, He released a spirit of hope which is an emotional force; and it forms the emotional component in relevant communications about hope. This Scripture shows that this spirit of hope is a form of grace from God for people to have a brighter future outlook in this dead and dying natural realm. Hope gives us something on which to anchor our future. Without this strong spirit of hope many would give up in despair. When we have a spirit of hope, it is not that we are reasoning our way to hope. Instead, God sends the spiritual force of hope as an emotional mantle to cover and calm us. It gives us the energy and power to wait in faith for God's promises to be fulfilled. Men without God have no spirit of hope covering them. People in a weak relationship with God will have less of the spirit of hope.

Romans 8:24

²⁴ For we are saved by hope: but hope that is seen is not hope: for what a man seeth, why doth he yet hope for?

This Scripture shows that hope for salvation is a driving emotional force to keep us looking for salvation until it arrives. When the salvation comes, then we no longer need to keep focused and encouraged by the spirit of hope.

Romans 15:13

¹³ Now the God of hope fill you with all joy and peace in believing, that ye may abound in hope, through the power of the Holy Ghost.

This Scripture shows us that God is the God of hope (no other god is a god of hope). The power of hope is a spiritual emotion with considerable energy released as part of the ministry of the Holy Spirit.

Galatians 5:5

[5] For we through the Spirit wait for the hope of righteousness by faith.

It is the Holy Spirit who gives us the energy to wait until we are redeemed, as the Lord Jesus Christ provides a cover of righteousness to us when we accept Him as a substitute for our sins and confess Him to be our Lord and Savior.

2 Thessalonians 2:16

[16] Now our Lord Jesus Christ himself, and God, even our Father, which hath loved us, and hath given *us* everlasting consolation and good hope through grace.

We are given a spirit of hope to sustain us in adversity until the promise of God comes. Hope is a spirit that is a part of the more powerful Spirit of Grace, which is one of the foundational Seven Spirits of God.

1 Peter 1:21

[21] Who by him do believe in God, that raised him up from the dead, and gave him glory; that your faith and hope might be in God.

This Scripture affirms that it is the Lord Jesus Christ who is the answer God has to anyone who wants to know who God is.

Conclusion about the nature of hope

We can conclude that the emotion of hope is a grace given to men by God to sustain them in adverse circumstances until the promises of God become manifest. It is a part of the Spirit of Grace.

Defining Faith

The two Scriptures below show God's answer as to what faith is.

Romans 10:17

[17] So then faith *cometh* by hearing, and hearing by the word [*rhema*] of God.

In the verse above *rhema* indicates a spoken utterance. We obtain faith by hearing the Lord God speak to us in an individual utterance. The Holy Spirit may speak the utterance by highlighting a part of Scripture. Faith is never a corporate blessing, although often men use the concept that way. God may speak the same message to many people at the same time; and in this sense it would become corporate.

Thus, faith comes when one believes what God speaks to him individually. In this sense it gives one the basis to hope for the coming forth of the word spoken by God throughout various adversities. This is the message in the Scripture below. One has to become comfortable separating God's communications in his heart from other communications (Hebrews 4:12). This comes by experience (by reason of use [Hebrews 5:14]).

Hebrews 11:1

[1] Now faith is the substance of things hoped for, the evidence of things not seen.

Once we see a thing, we no longer have to trust God for it. Also we no longer have to keep hoping for it, since it has arrived.

Belief in the Heart

Having "belief in the heart" is a foundational requirement for the fulfillment of many promises made by God to men. We are going to lay a foundation to develop what "belief in the heart" is. Mark 11:23-24 is a passgage which emphasizes this need.

Mark 11:23–24

[23] For verily I say unto you, That whosoever shall say unto this mountain, Be thou removed, and be thou cast into the sea; and shall not doubt in his heart, but shall believe that those things which he saith shall come to pass; he shall have whatsoever he saith. [24] Therefore I say unto you, What things soever ye desire, when ye pray, believe that ye receive *them*, and ye shall have *them*.

We need to understand the difference between belief in the heart and belief in the mind of the soul. What we believe in the heart is how we, how God, and how the demonic powers see the content of our heart. This is why the content of the heart is such a critical issue. It is what wins and loses spiritual wars with evil agents.

We are going to spend some time looking at this, because it is a very important issue; and it is frequently not understood.

The Sovereignty of God versus the free choice of man to decide his own course

In our book *How to be Led by the Spirit of God: Maturing in the Spirit* in Chapter 10 we listed 45 Scriptures indicating different things that God can do and that God has done to the heart of a person. If God decides for His overall purposes for history that a particular person must change his heart, then God can and will sovereignly change it (with or without the person's agreement). In these Scriptures we see God hardening hearts, softening hearts, and placing various words in them. When terms such as *hardening* and *softening* are used, they are relative to how a person decides to deal with God's words and instructions. All of the inclinations of a person's heart, as described in Scripture, are related to his beliefs and attitudes toward God.

When God was dealing with Pharaoh in the time of Moses, many times He hardened Pharaoh's heart. However, Pharaoh also hardened his own heart.

Exodus 8:32 and 9:12 relate some of these actions (which occurred many times).

Exodus 8:32

[32] And Pharaoh hardened his heart at this time also, neither would he let the people go.

Exodus 9:12

[12] And the LORD hardened the heart of Pharaoh, and he hearkened not unto them; as the LORD had spoken unto Moses.

There are many Scriptures indicating that God hardened the hearts of the children of Israel; but there are also some which indicate that they hardened their own hearts.

The authors believe that God will never take away the only real choice that a person has in life, the choice of where he will spend the eternal ages. The choices are to be with God or not to be with God. The Scripture below states that God will build circumstances into every person's life to allow him to go on the path that he has chosen. There is always room, until a final point known only to God occurs, for any person to go in the opposite direction.

Proverbs 16:9

[9] A man's heart deviseth his way: but the LORD directeth his steps.

We see, therefore, that God will allow a person to build spiritual structures in his heart that coincide with his choices. We will continue to look further into what belief in the heart means in the next section.

Thoughts in the Mind and in the Heart

The thoughts in the mind are transient and do not have much of a structure to support them. They come and go between the minds of the soul, the flesh, the inner man, and the heart. There is a memory in all four minds, but it is in the heart where thoughts are organized and stored into organized structures (high places, idols, tables, imaginations (always future oriented), attitudes, and beliefs). In addition, there can be evil spirits influencing the heart. After the second birth the Holy Spirit and the Law of God are present in the heart. As one deepens his relationship with God and his heart is strengthened (Ephesians 3:16-17), the Lord Jesus will also dwell in the heart.

People meditate in both their mind of the soul and the heart, and these thoughts go back and forth between the two minds (Romans 2:15). People ponder in their heart. The heart is deep, and a person does not know everything that he has stored in his heart (things can be hidden). The structures which one builds over time and the spiritual city which he forms determine how other spiritual beings see him.

The essential difference between the thoughts in the mind of the soul and in the heart is the structure that is organized around them. It takes a while to build a structure, and the structure can be built of various materials and in various soils. Structures are not quickly changed. They require a considerable amount of force and time to change them. Building materials include the Word of God, experience, the word of demons, and the word of influential situations and people. Repeated patterns of experience tend to lead to larger structures. Building on the rock of God's Word leads to stronger structures.

To take a thought from the mind that is novel to the person and to get that thought formed into a structure in the heart are not easy. There are several ways to do it; only one is repetition. A lot depends on the power of the spirit conveying the thought and the state of the current structures in the heart—including materials with which they are built and soil on which they are built. Since many situations are already organized in structures in the heart, we will look only at novel situations.

We will shortly examine the buildings in the heart, looking at various features which will determine resisitance to change. These include the material with which they are made, the soil on which they are built, and any idols within them. Some structures are better able to resist spiritual forces that seek to demolish or change them better than others. Before looking at these things we will examine how to change the heart and some spiritual conditions which make it hard to change the heart.

Changing the heart

Changing a city from one spiritual state to another involves using a powerful force acting over sufficient time to overcome those forces within it which resist the change. Sometimes a key weakness can be identified and exploited (an Achilles' heel), using a less powerful force over a shorter time. The four factors to assess in attempting change are the following: to identify any key weaknesses using spiritual discernment and by probing defenses; to determine the spiritual powers present which will resist change (this will include demonic influence in behavior patterns such as one sees in addictions); to determine how well-organized and integrated with other structures the forces within a particular thought and behavior pattern are; and to determine what other forces for change may be present at a particular time (such as a recent bereavement or other emotional stress from a significant life event).

In order to change the heart and the content of it, one must have a spiritual force acting on the contents which is strong enough and which acts over a long enough time in order to overcome the current defense from the idols, high places, imaginations, and power from any evil spirits which might be present. Thus, a very powerful force might completely disrupt the content and defense, as happened with the apostles after meeting the risen Lord Jesus Christ and subsequently being filled with the Holy Spirit at Pentecost. One small force acting at a weak point in defenses may also lead to change. There are many combinations of change strategy versus defense. Some hearts are more exposed than others to novel thoughts and are softer and less resistant to new thoughts.

It is not easy to change the heart just by repetition unless there is a reasonable amount of power in the force being applied to try to bring about the change. God brings various forces into one's life in order to promote change. These forces may include exposure to new people with different ideas, allowing an illness, inducing work place issues, and many more possibilities.

The term hardness of heart is a common concept in Scripture. It is a quality that resists change by failure to recognize, meditate on, and otherwise deal with new spiritual-realm material that is presented to one's natural senses. Scripture uses the term to denote the presence of a negative force toward being influenced by the actions of God. Such actions include the miracles. We will look at how the disciples dealt with seeing some of the miracles.

Discerning if one believes something in his heart

There are many people who have heard that one has to believe in the heart for that belief to be acceptable to God. They become concerned about how they can know when they have a belief in the heart, as opposed to having it just in the mind.

The thoughts of the mind are transient and fleeting. In any discussion one may hear many thoughts with which he can agree. This does not mean that he will ever act on them in any significant life .situations. He may agree that it is a good stock market but that does not mean he will invest in it. He may agree that the Lord Jesus Christ rose from death but this does not mean that he has placed his life in trusting this for eternal salvation. The thoughts of the heart are organized into structures about life situations and concepts important to each person.

Those things which we believe in our heart are those things on which we actually act. If we are not sure about what we believe in our heart then we can consider what we would do in an emergency. This is not a universally reliable test but can be helpful.

We know that recurring thoughts in the mind have been established as a belief concept in our heart when we act without thinking to the same information with the same behavioral response. A trivial example would be buying the same toothpaste when supplies are low. A spiritual example would be to defend creation against evolution regardless of the circumstances. If we have to consider circumstances for defending creation, then the belief has not matured into a spiritually mature concept, since it is based on what man thinks of us and not what God thinks of us. Regardless of how strong our beliefs in the heart are the devil may try to place in the mind a doubt against them, which must be dismissed summarily from the mind.

Only those beliefs which are built on a very extensive base of well integrated and organized Scripture surrounding a theme (such as healing) will be impregnable from attack by the demons. If we do not have a relevant Scripture organized into the overall understanding God provides in His Word related to healing, the demons will be able to exploit those things which we believe but which are not true. It has taken many years for us to get to this position on divine healing.

The Biblical teaching on the authority of a believer is a narrow topic and pondering it may help one to understand how to build a base of truth in his heart from which he can act. It is wise to know when and if one can take authority over demonic forces. If one does not use his authority when he has been given it, he wastes time and resources. If one attempts to use authority he does not have from God, evil spirits could injure him. One should never ever walk beyond his faith and what he believes firmly in his heart; to do so is regarded as sin by God and involves at the least a presumption on God to defend him.

Hardness of Heart

Hardness of heart is a spiritual illness which has a profound impact on people and on the ability to receive spiritual-realm wisdom, understanding, and knowledge.

It is rooted in sin. This is usually not a headline-grabbing sin, and most of the time it is being disobedient to God's speaking to one. The Scriptures below discuss hardness of heart. Hebrews 3:15 directly links the ability to hear God properly with hardening one's heart which comes from chronic sin patterns.

Hebrews 3:13

[13] But exhort one another daily, while it is called To day; lest any of you be hardened through the deceitfulness of sin.

Hebrews 3:15

[15] While it is said, To day if ye will hear his voice, harden not your hearts, as in the provocation.

Hardness of heart is a spiritual condition, rooted in sin, which, based on the Scriptures below, makes it very difficult for natural-realm observations to impact the spiritual understanding. The three Scriptures below show this.

Mark 6:52

[52] For they considered not *the miracle* of the loaves: for their heart was hardened.

The apostles had seen the miracle of feeding the multitudes and yet were still astonished and frightened to see the Lord Jesus Christ walking on water. They had failed to consider or meditate upon the meaning of the miracles they had observed, which showed the great control the Lord Jesus Christ had over the natural realm. The hardness of their hearts had made them unable to process the miraculous events they had witnessed into a new understanding of the creation and into an understanding of the Lord Jesus Christ and His power over the natural realm. The Lord Jesus Christ made the diagnosis so we can rule out that they had just an inability to process the new information due to intellectual challenge. It was a defense of the self-image which did not want to have to make the huge changes that true acknowledgement of the miracle-working power demanded.

We can all use this same test the Lord Jesus Christ used to diagnose hardness of heart in His apostles. Ponder how much the miraculous events we have heard of and read of influence our daily behavior. If a person cannot readily discuss tmiraculous events of which he has heard and point to tangible behavioral changes he has made, then the diagnosis is obvious. If he has not pondered the miracles at all, then there is a second spiritual illness of disobedience to God present; for He asks us to meditate upon His Word and to do this continually.

Mark 10:5

[5] And Jesus answered and said unto them, For the hardness of your heart he wrote you this precept.

This Scripture shows that God allowed Moses to modify His laws because of the insensitivity of the hearts of the Israelites to the spiritual issues surrounding divorce. They refused to process in their hearts that God required something new of them. Divorce is not something that God condones at all. He allows it in only a few circumstances. While divorce has obvious natural realm issues, it has even more profound impact on the spirit and on the spiritual realm.

Mark 16:14

[14] Afterward he appeared unto the eleven as they sat at meat, and upbraided them with their unbelief and hardness of heart, because they believed not them which had seen him after he was risen.

This Scripture shows that when a heart is hard, even amazing information given by trusted people and friends does not get through the heart to the mind of the soul in order to impact decision making.

For many people these days hardness of heart develops when one accepts false wisdom, understanding, and knowledge of the world system as truth. When one even pretends to hold these as correct, he is denying the truth of the Scripture. If one bases behavior on these false world system philosophies, he is living a lie. This is why hardness of heart so often involves suppressing and denying spiritual-realm reality. The person just does not want to see spiritual truth and reality for many reasons—perhaps to protect a job or to protect social standing. This is not the same as accepting that the world system believes falsehood but still working in it. It is imperative that one must gently and kindly stand against it when he has to choose between standing up for God or promoting a lie. One clearly has to stand up for the Lord; otherwise He will deny him. It is a matter of being *in* the world but not *of* it (1 John 2:15).

Summary

In summary, hardness of the heart is a spiritual block to natural-realm events being processed as evidence of spiritual realm reality, usually to protect something of value. Each time in the above Scriptures the information did not lead to appropriate changes in understanding and behavior. In the healthy spiritual heart one should be seeing the evidence of God's actions in organizing all of the natural realm events for His purposes. In the cases above this did not happen. The minds of the apostles had not been renewed to place the spiritual-realm functioning as foundational to the functioning of the natural realm.

Hardness of heart comes when one maintains chronic sinful beliefs and attitudes of which he has never repented. When a person believes in the heory of evolution this is strong evidence of hardness of heart. When someone tries to compromise and accept abortion, then this will lead to hardening of the heart; abortion breaks many of the commandments, including the first commandment God gave mankind.

The power that changed the hearts of the apostles

Thomas would not even believe the other ten apostles when they told him of their encounter with the risen Lord Jesus Christ; but when the risen Lord Jesus Christ appeared to him also, then he believed. The presence of the risen Lord Jesus Christ with the apostles several times softened the hearts of the apostles. There were power and authority in the risen Lord which would have been palpable to these apostles. This spiritual realm power was more than sufficient to overcome the hardness of their hearts. The apostles were able to keep the commandment in the Scripture below.

Matthew 28:18–20

[18] And Jesus came and spake unto them, saying, All power is given unto me in heaven and in earth. [19] Go ye therefore, and teach all nations, baptizing them in the name of the Father, and of the Son, and of the Holy Ghost: [20] Teaching them to observe all things whatsoever I have commanded you: and, lo, I am with you alway, *even* unto the end of the world. Amen.

The apostles were literally forced by this huge spiritual powerinto new behaviors, which continued to remold the structures in their hearts. The incredible power unleashed on the apostles at Pentecost also reshaped the structures in their hearts, and the hardness was gone. Frequently, God gives people time to allow Him to work more gently to remake the structures in the heart to be conducive to spiritual growth and spiritual-realm service. Look at the passage below.

Romans 2:3–5

[3] And thinkest thou this, O man, that judgest them which do such things, and doest the same, that thou shalt escape the judgment of God? [4] Or despisest thou the riches of his goodness and forbearance and longsuffering; not knowing that the goodness of God leadeth thee to repentance? [5] But after thy hardness and impenitent heart treasurest up unto thyself wrath against the day of wrath and revelation of the righteous judgment of God.

This Scripture shows that hardness of heart, coupled with an unwillingness to repent (which involves change), will ultimately lead to eternal separation from God. There are many spiritual illnesses which cause problems with the normal and proper function of the spiritual heart as God designed it to work.

Spiritual blindness and deafness

Spiritual blindness and spiritual deafness are other spiritual illnesses which result from a heart that is sinful.

Ephesians 4:18

[18] Having the understanding darkened, being alienated from the life of God through the ignorance that is in them, because of the blindness of their heart:

Matthew 13:15

[15] For this people's heart is waxed gross, and *their* ears are dull of hearing, and their eyes they have closed; lest at any time they should see with *their* eyes, and hear with *their* ears, and should understand with *their* heart, and should be converted, and I should heal them.

These Scriptures show that people are able to block any perception of a spiritual-realm cause behind natural-realm phenomena. The people wanted to defend their current self-image and the associated lifestyles. They did not want to be healed.

The Structures and the soil in the heart

We will now look at the types of material with which the spiritual structures in the heart are built and the soils on which they are built

God's ideal condition for the spiritual heart

God's ideal for the condition of the spiritual heart is for the soul to have been through the second birth; to have a new spirit which is clean and healthy; to have a pure heart in which the Holy Spirit dwells; and to have the image of the Lord Jesus Christ formed in the heart and in which the Father and the Son dwell.

The closer to the truth the image we form of the Lord Jesus Christ in the heart will determine how accurately we portray Him to other people. We need to know Him, His character, His abilities, and His power well; and we have to develop a balanced understanding of how and when He uses all of these attributes.

John 14:23

[23] Jesus answered and said unto him, If a man love me, he will keep my words: and my Father will love him, and we will come unto him, and make our abode with him.

Galatians 4:19

[19] My little children, of whom I travail in birth again until Christ be formed in you,

An individual must expend much spiritual energy and power to defeat the evil spirits and the flesh in order to reach this high ideal expressed in the two Scriptures above. God will willingly give it as He sees the energy used appropriately and not spent on any lusts of the flesh.

1 Thessalonians 5:23

[23] And the very God of peace sanctify you wholly; and *I pray God* your whole spirit and soul and body be preserved blameless unto the coming of our Lord Jesus Christ.

James 4:7

[7] Submit yourselves therefore to God. Resist the devil, and he will flee from you.

These two Scriptures above show that with God's help and power one can defeat the flesh and the demonic forces. To defeat the evil spirits, one must first submit to God in all things.

Structures in the Heart prior to the second birth

In our hearts we have high places, tables, imaginations, and idols prior to the second birth. On the high places we sacrifice our time and resources to our idols—clothing, cars, work, entertainment, and other similar. natural-realm attractions. After the second birth God will, as one submits his will to Him, erect fortresses, refuges, and strong towers. We have to let God work with us to take natural-realm wisdom, understanding, and knowledge out of our heart; remove idols; break down high places (these are the places we sacrifice to idols); eliminate wicked and self-promoting imaginations; and help us to obey all of His commands, including taking all thoughts captive.

Natural-Realm Structures in the heart

Natural realm structures are always built on false facts. It cannot be otherwise. Nonetheless, they can be strong and can be significant barriers to God. In the end, they are all built on sand; and when the end of this age comes, every knee will bow and every tongue will confess that Jesus Christ is Lord (Philippians 2:10-11).

The reason why these structures are relatively strong is that there has been poorly-contested repetitive indoctrination of philosophies and pseudo-religions, both promoted by the demonic powers through the world system education systems, and false religious systems which have varied through the history of this age. They remain strong because the Church has not been a strong adversary, having been dazzled in recent centuries by natural-realm science and technology.

These structures are built on widely held natural-realm philosophies and religions; they are supported by technological achievements built on natural-realm sciences. A highly visible miracle would bring these structures down (as happened in the wars between Israel and its enemies in the Old Testament era) were it not for the role of the flesh supporting them. The flesh partners with demonic philosophies to build itself up in pride. The pride is based on power, money, fame, and achievements. The combination of the flesh supporting the demonic philosophies to maintain its own status makes for strong barriers against the penetration of anything of God.

When a person has a strong interest to protect structures in the heart in order to preserve his position, then he will use a lot of self-deception to avoid a challenge. These mechanisms of deceiving oneself include all of the recognized psychological defense mechanisms. Ultimately, all of these defenses that individuals use are based on a lie. The flesh is relatively weak compared with demonic power ,and it has to have the power from the demonic philosophies which oppose God in all aspects in order to succeed, even temporarily.

All of these philosophies of demons and issues of the flesh are vain (empty) in the overall plans of God for the ages to come. They will all cease and will be shown as empty of anything of eternal worth. These philosophies and the pride of the flesh, if pursued, are a waste of a person's time and effort.

It is important for a child of God to learn natural-realm knowledge for the purpose of being able to hold a specific position in society. Daniel and his friends to do this (Daniel 1:4 and 1:20). When learning natural wisdom and knowledge, one must keep the overall perspective well in mind.

The Heart immediately after the second birth

Immediately after the second birth the heart is pure and new. There are no evil structures in it which are opposed to God. Since the mind is not renewed the heart will eventually be dominated by the flesh, unless there is rapid spiritual growth and maturation. Spiritual growth requires absorbing the Word of God and receiving the power of God, Even then the spirit grows only when the soul promotes it over the flesh. If the soul does not know how to mature his spirit by feeding on the Word, listening to and obeying God, and being strengthened by the power of God (and many churches do not teach this), then the new creation of God becomes a flesh-driven individual as were many in the Corinthian Church.

Within a few months this new man is little better than his contemporary who has not been through the second birth, except he does belong to God and will be of some help to God's plans. Such individuals build in their hearts structures of the flesh fed by world system thinking. The defenses against God are not nearly as strong as they are in the heart of a person who has not been given a second birth, since this soul has experienced God. He is aware of God and has been exposed in a small way to the spiritual realm. With good instruction he will quickly come to his proper place in God's Kingdom.

The vast majority of people in the Church in the West need a reconstruction in their hearts so that these new world system structures can be bulldozed. The individual then can work with God toward the ideal He wishes, which we discussed above. God wants His people to love Him and not to be drawn by fleshly lusts and desires. God wants relationship first; and then work for His Kingdom can flow from the relationship.

These people need a strong program of education, training, and mentoring. Such a program would need to teach the structure of man and how to use knowledge of this structure to identify resistant blocks in the heart. These blocks are caused by evil spirits supplying energy to various fleshly structures built in the heart. The demons use the flesh to distract the people into natural realm solutions.

The evil spirits will press their agenda to block the spiritual development of God's people through all of the power they have. They will try to confuse; they will try to make a soul doubt the character of God; they will try to keep a focus on the flesh through health issues; and they will try to stop people from communicating with God. They will try to keep people busy with natural-realm issues and diminish access to the Word of God through resource and time constraints. They will feed lusts, and these lead to sin which separates a soul from his God until repentance occurs (Isaiah 59:1-8 and Isaiah 64:5-7). All the sins mentioned in these Scriptures which separated God from His people have contemporary counterparts in the Church. The idols are different, but they are still false gods and consist of the fruits of mammon (money) in varied forms. God requires His people to repent before He will bless them.

The heart of a person who has been given a second birth after he realizes his heart needs purification

When a person realizes that his new heart has become impossibly impure and that his new spirit is unclean, he will want to embark on a program to correct these problems. If he is not careful, he might use fleshly thinking to make the corrections. This will not work. The corrections need to be made by God as the person commits to renewal of the mind and purification of the heart (discussed in Chapter 3). If God is not the author of the changes, then it will not be He who builds the new structures and who takes down the old structures.

Psalm 127:1

[1] Except the LORD build the house, they labour in vain that build it: except the LORD keep the city, the watchman waketh *but* in vain.

As one commits to God to pursue loving Him as he should, obeying all of His commands, listening to Him, and performing His work at His direction then God will act. God will use Scripture to tear down those things which need to be disposed; He will alter the street plan of the city within the heart to suit His purposes; and He will start to build new structures that are built on His Word. He will start to build stores for His true wisdom, understanding, and knowledge.

We can tell the difference between true and false wisdom, understanding, and knowledge by how they fit with Scripture. This fit has to be revealed supernaturally through personal revelation of the meaning of various Scriptures. There may be a spirit of knowledge which just "clunks" into place in the spirit with a satisfying spiritual thud; a prophesy which tests true in the spirit; or an explanation of doctrine which has no taint of man's wisdom. In addition, God may cement these teachings with power to authenticate His giving them. These concepts will "bulldoze" old structures and lay foundations and structures for the new ones. God will build all His structures on the rock, and they will weather the storms of the spiritual attacks.

One can understand why the taking in of true wisdom, understanding, and knowledge has to be from the spirit and not from the flesh when one looks at the Pharisees. They had intensely studied Scripture, and yet they missed completely Who the Lord Jesus Christ is. Similarly, there are many seminaries in the West that teach theology from a fleshly academic position and entirely miss the understanding of spiritual revelation.

One has to discern what is coming from the spirit to the mind of the soul from all other thoughts coming into the mind of the soul. This comes by practice. By learning the way God the Holy Spirit communicates, one can be sure that an idea is from true wisdom, understanding, and knowledge. Discernment increases with practice and repetition (Hebrews 5:14).

Some Scriptures below help in understanding all of this.

2 Corinthians 7:1

[1] Having therefore these promises, dearly beloved, let us cleanse

ourselves from all filthiness of the flesh and spirit, perfecting holiness in the fear of God.

1 Corinthians 14:6

[6] Now, brethren, if I come unto you speaking with tongues, what shall I profit you, except I shall speak to you either by revelation, or by knowledge, or by prophesying, or by doctrine?

This Scripture mentions four ways one can receive spiritual wisdom, understanding, and knowledge. The fifth way is to see God using His power (1 Corinthians 2:4).

Matthew 7:24–27

[24] Therefore whosoever heareth these sayings of mine, and doeth them, I will liken him unto a wise man, which built his house upon a rock: [25] And the rain descended, and the floods came, and the winds blew, and beat upon that house; and it fell not: for it was founded upon a rock. [26] And every one that heareth these sayings of mine, and doeth them not, shall be likened unto a foolish man, which built his house upon the sand: [27] And the rain descended, and the floods came, and the winds blew, and beat upon that house; and it fell: and great was the fall of it.

God's plan for the city within the heart will be similar to the statement we made at the beginning of this section and which we repeat here.

God's ideal for the condition of the spiritual heart is for the soul to have been through the second birth, to have a new spirit which is clean and healthy, to have a pure heart in which the Holy Spirit dwells, to have the image of the Lord Jesus Christ formed in it, and to have the Father and the Son dwell in it.

We will now look at the two enemies of healing, the flesh and evil spirits.

Healing Hardness of Heart

One must consider how futile pursuit of the empty world system is for the short period one lives in it (at most 70 years). In return for gaining a short-term partial reward, he may sacrifice eternal rewards. He is in danger of God's condemning him to eternal separation from Him for disobedience. If one is chronically hard of heart, he should examine himself and question whether he has ever received the second birth. His hardness of heart will melt through repentance and a complete reversal of his beliefs, attitudes, and behavior so that he is actively renewing his mind, purifying his heart, and taking his thoughts captive.

In His kindness God will often bring a severe spiritual challenge, such as illness, in order to help a person examine himself and to meditate on truth. The heart sometimes requires severe challenges to the spirit to break the hardness of the heart.

2 Corinthians 13:5

[5] Examine yourselves, whether ye be in the faith; prove your own selves. Know ye not your own selves, how that Jesus Christ is in you, except ye be reprobates?

The Evil Spirits

God set up the creation so that there is a war between Him and the evil spirits for the hearts of men. It is little wonder that the devil acted against the first occupants of the earth, Adam and Eve. A major reason the devil is interested in harming men is to thwart God and thus to inflict suffering on God. He hates the image of God which is in man; thus, he tries to destroy this image with all of the means he has at his disposal. God created man with less power than the angels and evil spirits; but potentially man can have greater power as he relies on God to supply it. Few people even understand the nature of the war which evil spirits wage. Evil spirits can harm the flesh and will bring various diseases, infirmities, and illnesses. They can inflame fleshly lusts for power, fame, and wealth. (God sometimes gives these as gifts but not when the flesh lusts for them.) They promote pride and negative emotions—anger, jealousy greed, doubt (especially in God), envy, and hate. The evil spirits are not able to love, admire, praise truthfully, and be grateful. They are never meek or mild; have no kindness and no patience. They are clamorous and bellicose. The Scripture informs us that they have only three goals; it contrasts these with what the Lord Jesus Christ provides.

John 10:10

¹⁰ The thief cometh not, but for to steal, and to kill, and to destroy: I am come that they might have life, and that they might have *it* more abundantly.

The abundant life promised in the Scripture above by the Lord Jesus Christ comes as one is born into a whole new realm (it is not more of the same from the natural realm). There are new treasures and areas of interest in this new (to a person) and greater realm. There are fresh and stimulating challenges. There are difficulties, but there are great rewards for those who overcome them.

Victory over Evil Spirits

We looked earlier at the relative power of God over the devil and the evil spirits. The devil, Satan, can do nothing that the Lord God does not allow (Job 1). God uses the demonic forces in a sense to discipline and to get the attention of His children. The story of the plagues God placed on the Egyptians as told in the Exodus shows how God uses and controls evil spirits by placing boundaries on them. Also review. Pharaoh's magicians could not keep up with the miracles wrought by God through Moses.

Spirit never dies in the sense of a physical death (as occurs with the destruction of the flesh). The spirits of men, angels, and evil spirits live eternally. The only issue is in which abode they will live during the ages to come.

Luke 12:5

⁵ But I will forewarn you whom ye shall fear: Fear him, which after he hath killed hath power to cast into hell; yea, I say unto you, Fear him.

We know that spirits can be damaged; we know that the Lord bound some evil spirits before the Flood (Jude 6); and we know that the spirits believe that God will torment them eventually (Matthew 8:29). In Luke 12:5 above the Lord Jesus Christ is referring to killing the flesh of men. Very powerful spirits over geographic areas of influence cannot be killed, but the prayers of the saints can displace them. Francis Frangipane wrote about these issues. A spirit being with more power can displace them from their area of jurisdiction (Daniel 10:11-13). God's children, when they join in agreement in prayer, have a great multiplier impact in displacing spiritual powers, and more so as He gives more power to assist their prayers.

At the cross the Lord Jesus won the final victory over the devil. When we dwell in God's secret place (Psalm 91:1-6), then we already have victory over the demonic spirits. If we choose to step outside this protection, then we are vulnerable to attack. All sickness will be healed, and all demons will flee when we perform the following: strengthen ourselves in God and the power of His might, let Him fill our hearts with love, carry the image of the Lord Jesus Christ in our hearts, and have the Father and the Son abide with us. Few, if any people in the Church in the West reach this level of intimacy with God, and few will have His trust to perform the miracles this relationship would facilitate.

John 14:12

¹² Verily, verily, I say unto you, He that believeth on me, the works that I do shall he do also; and greater *works* than these shall he do; because I go unto my Father.

This Scripture gives the basis for what we just said above. To believe on the Lord Jesus Christ as described in this Scripture above, we have to know Him very well; or we might have some false ideas about Him and His character. We have to look carefully at such Scriptures. The word *believeth* would means "believe in the heart"; although this is not stated in this particular Scripture.

When we carry the presence of the Lord with u,s then the demons will fear and tremble because of Him (not because of us). This is the impact the presence of the Lord has on demonic spirits. Many of the healing miracles relate the contacts between the Lord Jesus Christ and demons. Many pleaded with Him for various purposes, but all had to obey Him.

James 2:19

[19] Thou believest that there is one God; thou doest well: the devils also believe, and tremble.

James 4:7

[7] Submit yourselves therefore to God. Resist the devil, and he will flee from you.

Resisting the devil in the context of James 4:6-8 indicates that we have to have true humility, as we see how small we are and how little we can do in comparison to how great God is and how much He can do. We have to have humility in the spirit, not just in fleshly acts. We then have to submit ourselves in all ways to God for being led by His Spirit (Romans 8:14). We also have to draw very close to God so that His presence and ours are merged. Then the devil will flee from us, but not because of who we are. He does, however, recognize spiritual giants (Acts 19:15).

Finally, Ephesians 6:10–18 explain how we need to live. This Scripture is extremely important; for if we fulfill it adequately, then we will be able to stand against the evil spirits at all times. We point out a few of the very important points in this Scripture below it.

[10] Finally, my brethren, be strong in the Lord, and in the power of his might. [11] Put on the whole armour of God, that ye may be able to stand against the wiles of the devil. [12] For we wrestle not against flesh and blood, but against principalities, against powers, against the rulers of the darkness of this world, against spiritual wickedness in high *places*. [13] Wherefore take unto you the whole armour of God, that ye may be able to withstand in the evil day, and having done all, to stand. [14] Stand therefore, having your loins girt about with truth, and having on the breastplate of righteousness; [15] And your feet shod with the preparation of the gospel of peace; [16] Above all, taking the shield of faith, wherewith ye shall be able to quench all the fiery darts of the wicked. [17] And take the helmet of salvation, and the sword of the Spirit, which is the word of God: [18] Praying always with all prayer and supplication in the Spirit, and watching thereunto with all perseverance and supplication for all saints;

Important points to note in this passage of Scripture which to allow us to stand against the devil and the evil spirits:

1. We have to be strong in the Lord (within His character and perfect will). We have to be confident in His covering us with His power. We have to be close to Him and know Him well. God, the demons, and we will see us as who we are in our heart.

2. We have to put on and keep on 24/7/365 all six parts of the armor (these are commands).

3. We have to realize that men are not our enemies, and we have to live and fight in the spiritual realm for our success to occur. No natural-realm thinking or knowledge will help.

4. Our only potentially offensive weapon is the sword, and we can defend with it only to the extent of our comfort with the entire Scripture. We should use it offensively only as God clearly directs.

5. We have to pray always in the spirit. This will be a mixture of four things—keeping our spirit in the Kingdom where we keep it righteous, joyful, and peaceful; persevering in prayer; praying in the spirit without ceasing; and praying in our prayer language and with our renewed intellect.

When we fulfill these things, we can be sure of the victory; but sadly there are few churches training their congregations for this kind of effort. As a result, the Church in the West is very weak. When the Church is weak, individuals are weak. In such circumstances, even if God were to heal us spiritually and physically, it would probably be lost very quickly from demonic counter attacks.

We should be encouraged that we can defeat these evil spirits; but we have to be sober minded and let God train us how to come into the position where we can win. One must never, ever, confuse a good natural intellect with the spiritual equivalent. The spiritual intellect depends on the strength of the relationship with God and has nothing to do with our fleshly gifting. We must always let God and His angels do the fighting, unless specifically otherwise directed; for the battle is always the Lord's.(1 Samuel 17:47). We must always be obedient to His instructions in all battles. We must never speak evil against any evil power, for God also created them (2 Peter 2:12).

Taking authority over evil spirits

Taking authority over an evil spirit causing a disease can bring healing. This is a special situation, as we discuss below.

God delegates various levels of authority to each of His children (Luke 9:1) on a very individual basis so that one can perform the work to which God has called him. A small number of people will have the authority to command evil spirits and can expect acquiescence to his order (Luke 19:12-27 and Titus 2:15).

Such a person can confidently perform this without a special request to God for specific power in a particular situation. If one has this authority delegated, he will be aware of it. If he does not and is facing a demonic attack, he can ask God to increase the might in his spirit to defeat the enemy. God may grant this, and the person will be aware of his request's being granted (Ephesians 3:16).

If neither of these situations is present, one can ask people to pray with him for victory against a demonic attack (Matthew 18:19). It is essential if this is to succeed to get only those who believe in their heart the Scripture regarding the multiplication effect of two or more joining together in prayer (and such people may be very difficult to find).

If none of the above remedies is available one should always recall that the battle is the Lord's (1 Samuel 17:47),; and if one eliminates all sin patterns and draws close to God he can expect God to act on his behalf. God is constrained by His Word not to act if the individual has opened himself to an attack by his own previous decisions, until he repents (changes his mind, proceeds in the opposite direction, and seeks God's forgiveness).

Continuing Sin Patterns are enemies of healing.

A continuing sin pattern(s) will weaken us when we request healing. These are spiritual diseases, and we can ask God to strengthen him in the spirit to stand against these areas of weakness. We will look at some relevant Scriptures.

1 John 1:9

[9] If we confess our sins, he is faithful and just to forgive us *our* sins, and to cleanse us from all unrighteousness.

If we confess our sin problems to God and are sincerely and honestly seeking cleansing, He will not only forgive those sins of which we are aware; but He will also cleanse us from all of those of which we are not aware. This is a wonderful promise given to us in love. The next Scripture is very important when we approach God for healing. It deals with belief in our heart. If our heart is pure before God, then it will not condemn us; and we can have confidence for healing from God when we request it. Of course, there may be a timing issue.

1 John 3:19–21

[19] And hereby we know that we are of the truth, and shall assure our hearts before him. [20] For if our heart condemn us, God is greater than our heart, and knoweth all things. [21] Beloved, if our heart condemn us not, *then* have we confidence toward God.

If we have unconfessed sin (even if we are not completely aware of it or of what the issues are before God), we will have no confidence or assurance that God will heal us when we request it. This is the impact of sin on the heart. One cannot overcome this weakening impact through any fleshly effort. Just as Adam and Eve tried to hide from God after their sin, our heart and our flesh will try to hide from God; and will not be able to stand before Him. Anyone who is not confident that God will heal him needs to examine all of the causes of this lack of confidence. There are many—not understanding Scripture properly; being subject to evil spirits causing confusion; not knowing how to hear God (spiritual deafness); and unconfessed prior sins, which will block communication with God. There are many others but these are areas in which to look. unconfessed prior sins which will block communication with God

Love

There is one final tool which one can use to defeat evil spirits, that of having God's love in our heart. This is accessible to all, but it takes a very close relationship with God for this to be available to us. We will discuss it further later in this chapter. Being filled with God's love will bring spiritual healing by casting out all fear. We will know when we are filled with God's love when we experience it in a palpable way that is much more than intellectual understanding of the concept of love, but in a way that is deep and broad in the heart. We have to have God's love flowing through us. No evil spirits tolerate it, and they will leave voluntarily as the Scripture shows.

The Flesh

We have previously discussed what the Scriptures refer to under the term *flesh*. The flesh is all of the physical components of man. These include muscles, nerves, brain, organs, skin, bones, tendons, blood, and all other components. A fleshly mind is one that operates under the influence of the flesh and makes its decisions based on the influence of the flesh. The brain is not particularly fleshlier than any other component, but the term fleshly mind is related to the source of its memories, beliefs, attitudes, thinking, and thought processes.

A spiritual heart that is fleshly is one that operates under the influence of the flesh as it was before a second birth. All of the structures in it—all of the imaginations, desires, lusts, beliefs, attitudes, and emotions—are based on the satisfying of the flesh. It cannot be changed from being fleshly, except it be replaced at the time of the second birth.

God entirely rejected the flesh at the time Adam and Eve disobeying Him. At that time He judged it and sentenced it to eternal destruction and sentenced it to return to the dust from where it came. This disobedience was the original sin.

There are three major divisions into which sins of the flesh fall. These are shown in the scripture below.

1 John 2:16

[16] For all that *is* in the world, the lust of the flesh, and the lust of the eyes, and the pride of life, is not of the Father, but is of the world.

These sin patterns in God's eyes are really all that is in this world; and none of it is of God. It is interesting to note that the original sin fell into all three of these categories, and many sinful acts do.

Genesis 3:6

[6] And when the woman saw that the tree *was* good for food, and that it *was* pleasant to the eyes, and a tree to be desired to make *one* wise, she took of the fruit thereof, and did eat, and gave also unto her husband with her; and he did eat.

Eve saw with her eyes (lust of the eyes) that the tree was good for food (lust of the flesh). In addition she desired the fruit to make her wise (pride of life).

There are some sins God hates more than others. A Hebrew idiom indicates that the seventh, sowing discord among brethren, is the worst. God highly and greatly values unity of spirit. In this list three of the sins are mental attitude sins; three are sins of the tongue; only one (murder) is an overt action.

Proverbs 6:16–19

[16] These six *things* doth the LORD hate: yea, seven *are* an abomination unto him: [17] A proud look, a lying tongue, and hands that shed innocent blood, [18] An heart that deviseth wicked imaginations, feet that be swift in running to mischief, [19] A false witness *that* speaketh lies, and he that soweth discord among brethren.

Pride makes a man depend on his natural-realm skills; and even if he has gone through the second birth and has not appreciably renewed his mind, it will be hard not to leverage these skills into the spiritual realm. Pride is the basis of all discord (Proverbs 13:10).

Proverbs 13:10

[10] Only by pride cometh contention: but with the well advised *is* wisdom.

Winning a war against the flesh

This war is won step by step, as the new spirit is stronger than the flesh. The soul has to learn to suppress the impulses, lusts, and desires of the flesh and instead promote the desires of the spirit (Galatians 5:18). The flesh will never go away so this is a continual war. However, as the soul sows to the spirit, the flesh will weaken; and the fight will become easier. We have discussed the following cycle before. We take thoughts captive continually, renew the mind, and purify the heart. Eventually, the flesh can be made to serve the Lord God, as our spirit grows stronger (Romans 12:1).

Galatians 6:8

[8] For he that soweth to his flesh shall of the flesh reap corruption; but he that soweth to the Spirit shall of the Spirit reap life everlasting.

Romans 8:13

[13] For if ye live after the flesh, ye shall die: but if ye through the Spirit do mortify the deeds of the body, ye shall live.

Romans 12:1

[1] I beseech you therefore, brethren, by the mercies of God, that ye present your bodies a living sacrifice, holy, acceptable unto God, *which is* your reasonable service.

The combination of flesh and spirit

The flesh alone is powerful in opposing the new spirit. When evil spirits use it in their war against God, it has even more spiritual power to resist the new spirit. These spirits lend their power to the flesh. It is reassuring to note that as God places His power to strengthen one's spirit (Ephesian 3:16), the flesh and the spirits together will not prevail in any war, although the skirmish may last a while. We have seen that there is a hierarchy of evil spirits (Ephesians 6:12). One suspects these evil spirit rulers have one or more spirits appointed to try to vex each person in the world; probably more are appointed to those who have been through the second birth. Evil spirits are very common; the authors have noted atmospheres of various shades of depression over towns and cities in which they have lived and to which they have travelled (Ephesians 2:2—powers of the air). One of us spoke with medical missionaries to India, who recalled the heaviness of the atmosphere and who stated they would hear spirits thudding on the roof of the house.

All our thoughts are transparent to God and are relatively open to evil spirits. We do know that evil spirits are frequently wrong in the conclusions they draw and that they were completely out-maneuvered by the crucifixion of the Lord Jesus Christ. However, one would be safe to assume that they can make strongly-based inferences about what a person is thinking and planning. A lot of this may be based on intelligent associations. Bruce first started to realize some of this while practicing medicine. He noted that each time he saw a patient with a bad 'flu or cold, he had a picture in his mind of coming down with a similar problem. Usually that did not occur, but occasionally it did. Asking rhetorically why this happens led Bruce to a long search into demonic activity and how people are subliminally influenced in their thoughts by evil spirits. This has nothing to do with demonic possession, which is a real issue; we have seen it, but it is quite rare in our experience.

Demons frequently attack us by injecting thoughts, sometimes appropriately to what we are contemplating. More frequently, they try to influence future behavior by reminding us of past situations and imaginations.

They attack the flesh with illnesses; they attack by inducing lusts; and they attack by appealing to our pride of life (a new car, a better cell phone, and many other things).

Evil spirits tend to be clamorous and apply pressure. God never behaves in these ways. They tend to have noisy voices (occasionally screaming or shouting), and the thought content and the emotions are associated with negative emotions, espcially fear. These thoughts will keep coming back repetitively. At times these spirits will attempt to be intrusive. There is frequently an attempt to intimidate and accelerate hasty decision making due to a strong sense of fear. They are thoughts which one would easily put down to just his own imagination. (They are not thoughts that are intense and persecutory to the point of being disabling as is the case in psychiatric conditions.) All people are subject to these types of thoughts. The fears are related to being late, not having enough money, losing a job, being late for lunch, not appearing appropriately well dressed to the situation, not being successful on an exam, and many similar thoughts. Frequently the spirits will try to inflame lusts of all types by injecting thoughts to accelerate a situation. They are able to cause false symptoms and signs of illness, as we discuss below.

What these demons are trying to accomplish is to:

1. Have a person follow their agenda and not try to discern God's agenda, and

2. Make a person get into a sinful situation.

Then these same spirits turn around and accuse the individual to God and are successful. God does not condone following any spirit other than Him.

False symptoms and signs

The demonic spirits can inflict clinical signs in the flesh of a person. They will do this in an attempt to cause a person to believe he is ill. If one takes this bait and believes it, then he is following that spirit and not God. God is not pleased by this. God assures us that He will not allow a demon (or circumstance) to tempt one above his ability to withstand the temptation (1 Corinthians 10:13). As one grows in spiritual maturity and power, God might allow a demon to induce a false symptom in order that He might work good for His child. This type of attack, when overcome, will strengthen a person in his faith and belief. One should not expect God to allow this type of attack until he is very seasoned in the area of illness and demonic attacks. If he is not seasoned in this area and develops a symptom, then it is wiser for him to seek medical help, especially in any urgent situation. Most of the time it is more likely to be an illness based on natural-realm cause and effect laws. He could also seek sound counsel from his spiritual advisor. If he does not have a spiritual advisor who is seasoned in this area, then he should seek medical help.

Spiritual Communications from one spirit to another

All spiritual beings, including man, have a spirit which radiates a certain amount of spiritual power continually. When a spiritual being acts in any way, including communicating with another spirit being, it releases a spiritual flow consisting of information, emotion, and power. The intensity of each of these three aspects of the spirit can vary. What evil spirits like to do to intimidate is to attack a person with a strongly negative emotional force; and they will try to make the person associate this emotion he experiences with a particular situation. An example would be that of a spirit which carries an ability to transmit the emotion of jealousy (Numbers 5:14), attacking a person with a powerful emotional feeling of jealousy, inducing an emotion of jealousy in the person attacked. The evil spirit might contrive to do it at such a time as to have the victim associate this emotion with a person or a situation. These evil spirits are constantly attacking; usually people do not take any action and just dismiss the thoughts. However if only one percent of these attacks stick, then over time a lot of harm could be done to a person. This kind of thing is going on continually in our lives. Even if we understand the principle, we still have to be alert and vigilant to take his thoughts captive for Christ. These spirits do not readily flee. One has to mature to the point at which his spirit has increased in power. He also may have to ask God to give him further power in order to make them flee.

Evil spirits may enrage someone against a person without a rational basis. They will try to incite hatred, anger, and physical aggression toward other people. There are no limits to their evil.

These spirits try to interrupt communications with God by bringing thought patterns to people who have been through the second birth and who are not renewing their minds. These spirits well know that if a person fails to forgive it will block communications with God. Not loving one's spouse will do the same. There are many other sin patterns that, if continued, will interrupt the ability to hear God speak; and there are many current sin patterns in people in the Church (many sins of omission) which will cause God not to listen to a person (Isaiah 59:1-2 and 64:7). These spirits try to create these breaks in communication between a child of God and God. We have to build structures in our heart, as God directs, to bolster weaknesses which we can identify where the enemy makes continual attacks; and we have to build the image of our Lord, in our hearts (always with God's direction).

Doubt and false guilt

Two particularly disruptive emotions that a person who is a child of God may face and which he must learn to diagnose through analyzing the spirits in his thoughts are those of false guilt and doubt. False guilt stops a person following a path God may want him to follow. The emotion of doubt, when injected into the mind as a thought, is a treacherous way to try to interfere in the forming of trust in God, building faith, and building structures in the heart.

Matthew 21:21

[21] Jesus answered and said unto them, Verily I say unto you, If ye have faith, and doubt not, ye shall not only do this *which is done* to the fig tree, but also if ye shall say unto this mountain, Be thou removed, and be thou cast into the sea; it shall be done.

When we look at the Scripture above, the Lord Jesus Christ says to have faith (which comes from hearing him speak to a person about a particular action He wants done). We will learn through repetition how to know and separate His communications to us from those of our own imagination and from evil spirits. He then says not to doubt; so evil spirits, when they know God wants an individual to take a course of action will try to induce an emotion of doubt associated with the situation. If we quickly refute such a spirit, no harm is done; but these spirits will keep trying to induce doubt. However, if we start to doubt that God has spoken to us, then real harm is done to the relationship between God and us.

Familial Spirits

If there are illnesses which run in one's family one must at least ask about curses in the family. These curses are broken by the second birth which takes one into a new family. The spirits may still try to place a particular illness on a person without any right to do so. They always lie. One may have to make declarations and defend with a well-written declaration based on the Word of God and declared aloud. A lot of these battles can be protracted; but one can, with God's leadership, prevail in all cases. When one is in battle (all children of God are), then learning how to communicate with his commander (God) and doing so are critically important for his safety and for him to prevail in the skirmishes.

The war between the two kingdoms

We discussed this war extensively in our book *Spirit*. Some highlights follow. The demonic forces, well organized (Ephesians 6:12) into a hierarchical system which integrates with men, wage a constant war against God. It is a war against truth which is a fundamental element of God's character. The press and other literature use terms such as "post-truth" to describe our current society in the West.

The purposes of these evil spirits in this age are simply to prevent men reconciling to God and then from coming into a personal relationship with Him in which they are developed in the spiritual realm. They use many lines of attack to do this. The evil spirits highly personalize these attacks against each individual based on what he currently believes about God and the spiritual realm. If the first line of attack does not succeed, they will proceed to another. Some lines of attack are listed below. These lines all are designed to deny the existence of truth (God is truth), and, if that fails, to distort the nature of truth.

1. They will try to persuade men that God does not exist and that there is no spiritual realm.

2. They will portray God as distant and not interested in individuals.

3. They will distort all aspects of the character of God.

4. They will distort the nature of the second birth.

5. They will try to prevent a person's reaching any degree of spiritual maturity.

This war can be won only when individuals within the Church and the organized Church declare truth as it is in the spiritual realm. The secularized church is not winning this war, and a secularized church cannot win this war. We discuss this in the Chapter 8.

Winning the war against evil spirits

We have already addressed how to win the war against evil spirits, but it cannot be stressed enough. We have to be in a very close relationship with God and under His protective cover by keeping obedient to Him always. All men are in a constant war with evil spirits, which intensifies as one shows interest in the second birth. After the second birth it gets even more intense; and even worse as one tries to develop in power and wisdom in the spirit. That is why God is so pleased with those who overcome; to these people there are many wonderful promises.

People can always win this war and the many skirmishes, as we discussed above.

1. It is critical to change what we believe in the heart and to have confidence in God. We have to have an image in our hearts that we will win because of the presence of the

Lord and because of His character. Our heart must not be weakened by sin, but rather must be pure.

2. Keeping all of the armor on and well preserved as in Ephesians 6 is critical.

3.   There is additionally one other major effort we must make and that is to let the love of God fill us. We have to develop the capacity in our heart (with God) to accept it. When we do, the perfect love will cast out fear (fear is always demonic in origin). This love of God flowing through us will keep all evil spirits at bay. That in part is why pursuing love is so important to God. The Apostle John in his life on earth exemplified being filled with the love of God; he stressed it in his letters.

1 John 4:16–18

[16] And we have known and believed the love that God hath to us. God is love; and he that dwelleth in love dwelleth in God, and God in him. [17] Herein is our love made perfect, that we may have boldness in the day of judgment: because as he is, so are we in this world. [18] There is no fear in love; but perfect love casteth out fear: because fear hath torment. He that feareth is not made perfect in love.

We must come to a point of love in God where we have no fear because we see how great and powerful He is and how deeply He cares for us. We then dwell in God, and God dwells in us. That will keep all demons at bay. This position does not come cheaply. It does not come without much spiritual wrestling and struggle.

A place of rest

If we succeed in overcoming the devil through our relationship with God (there is no other way), we will enter into a period of rest, at least for a while, since the devil will depart from us. Hebrews 4:1-9 describes this rest.

¹ Let us therefore fear, lest, a promise being left *us* of entering into his rest, any of you should seem to come short of it. ² For unto us was the gospel preached, as well as unto them: but the word preached did not profit them, not being mixed with faith in them that heard *it*. ³ For we which have believed do enter into rest, as he said, As I have sworn in my wrath, if they shall enter into my rest: although the works were finished from the foundation of the world. ⁴ For he spake in a certain place of the seventh *day* on this wise, And God did rest the seventh day from all his works. ⁵ And in this *place* again, If they shall enter into my rest. ⁶ Seeing therefore it remaineth that some must enter therein, and they to whom it was first preached entered not in because of unbelief: ⁷ Again, he limiteth a certain day, saying in David, To day, after so long a time; as it is said, To day if ye will hear his voice, harden not your hearts. ⁸ For if Jesus had given them rest, then would he not afterward have spoken of another day. ⁹ There remaineth therefore a rest to the people of God.

We obtain this rest because we trust God, love God, and believe that we are loved by God. Therefore we cease from any need to do any work because we want to stay just in God's presence. At this point He will use us mightily for His Kingdom, but we will not be doing the work. His Spirit will carry us, energize us, direct us, and empower us.

Physical and Spiritual Healing

As we are filled with the Spirit of God and as we are a blessing to Him, we receive the promises of Psalm 103:1-5. Healing will come as our spirit is maturing, as our spiritual heart is purified, and as it is filled with the presence of God.

When one reads Psalm 103:1-2, it is obvious that King David, when talking about a person blessing God and His character with all that is within him, is speaking about a special manner of blessing God. It is equivalent to upholding the First Commandment and becoming closer to God. He then associates this with recalling God's benefits. God has let this association stand. In doing he connects the blessing of God with the receiving of these benefits. This allows us to make a very important point about the character of the Lord God. God is not guileful and would never allow any part of His Word to be not straightforward. He does hide things for us to search out, but this is not the same as being guileful. We should always read the Word with an expectation of the intent being straightforward. Scripture such as Isaiah 5:12 are literal in the spiritual realm and are not intended as allegory.

Emotional Healing

Many people carry wounds and scars in their hearts from early years. Many try to resolve these issues because of the concern that they continue to influence current health and emotional functioning negatively. Many seek counseling to help. Counseling can certainly help; but it frequently takes a long time and may be only partially successful. Usually counseling excludes much emphasis on the power to change the heart from the second birth. Counseling frequently uses natural-realm reasoning and thus omits addressing spiritual healing. The development of an ongoing and growing relationship with a God who displays true love and concern is the greatest healing one can obtain for early psychological injuries. As one focuses on growth in the spiritual realm, these early natural realm issues tend to recede in impact and importance. It is of paramount importance for a person to forgive those who have caused harm, for this is always a block to his healing. As one sees the person(s) who injured them from the perspective of God, the forgiving will become much easier. One should always work with his counselor and include discussion of the spiritual issues as appropriate. Having a deep and growing understanding of the spiritual realm will enable a person to see occasionally, as God opens His spiritual vision, the wicked forces that have been arrayed against those who injured him. This also makes forgiveness easier.

The Role of the Church

Most people attending the local church will not have been exposed to the teaching we have discussed in this book. This is not the way God wants His Kingdom to be operating; He wants the local church to equip His people for the war they are in so they can be victorious. He wants His people to grow in spiritual knowledge and understanding. The Scriptures below address these issues.

Ephesians 4:11–13

[11] And he gave some, apostles; and some, prophets; and some, evangelists; and some, pastors and teachers; [12] For the perfecting of the saints, for the work of the ministry, for the edifying of the body of Christ: [13] Till we all come in the unity of the faith, and of the knowledge of the Son of God, unto a perfect man, unto the measure of the stature of the fulness of Christ:

Our local churches are supposed to be bringing us to the stature in the spiritual realm of the fullness of the Lord Jesus Christ. That this is happening in very few churches in the West is grieving to God.

The Will of God for His Church is for Spiritual Healing.

Colossians 1:9

[9] For this cause we also, since the day we heard *it*, do not cease to pray for you, and to desire that ye might be filled with the knowledge of his will in all wisdom and spiritual understanding;

These desires, expressed in Colossians 1:9, also are not being fulfilled in the local churches. We think that God wants to bring a large correction to the churches in the West in the very near future. In a recent revelation of His will to Bruce, God revealed sixteen issues which have led to the current weakness in His Church. He does not want to discard the present Church and start in a new direction; this is never God's way since His very nature is to heal. God also revealed some things which have to be done to start this process of healing in the individuals within the churches and within the Church overall.

This book is about healing the individual members of God's family and God's character of healing. The condition of spiritual strength in the Church is very much a part of the combined strength of the individual members. There is a strong association between the spiritual health of the Church and the spiritual health of the individuals in it. Both need to be healed. Physical healing is associated with spiritual healing for individuals.

We need structures in the Church to provide education and assistance with nurturing and maturing members of the family of God in order to fulfill Ephesians 4:11–13 and Colossians 1:9.

We see fewer divine healings than should be the case. This is because of many structural issues in the current church in the West which have detached the Church from spiritual underpinnings into a more-realm mindset. The relative infrequency of church members seeking divine healing reflects this weakness. Many seem to prefer to seek healing within the respective medical systems in the various countries in the West. People pray for healing, but the impact of prayer and of its being answered by God is diluted by concurrent medical treatment. God expects those without faith in Him for healing to seek help from a physician and has provided this as a grace for society. It is sin to expect God to heal when there is not faith (Romans 14:23). The issue is that the churches have not fostered the development of faith.

In the next chapter we will discuss the things that God is indicating to be issues in His Church in the West and which have led to spiritual weakness and paucity. These impact the frequency and outcomes of divine healing of spiritual and physical problems.

The Healing of the Church

Chapter Eight

The Role of the Church in the securing of Divine Healing of the Members

The role of the Church overall, as the body of the Lord Jesus Christ on the earth, is to represent Him fully and to portray His Character; His promises to mankind; His power; His abilities; His method for making and operating the creation; the current state of man and of the creation; His expectations for the creation and how He designed man to fulfill them; His expectations of individuals; how to relate to Him; His purposes for the creation; and His future plans for the creation to those outside and inside the Church. As part of these charges the local churches are called to be salt and light to the society in ewhich they are operating. Understanding and receiving divine healing flow from these principles.

Healing and the Character of God

God's character is such that He must heal people to be true to who He is. His Words will never fail. Individuals and groups of people can prevent Him from healing by their attitudes, beliefs, and behaviors. Since the Lord Jesus Christ specifically paid for both sin and sickness in His suffering and crucifixion, His healing is available to all who call on Him in faith and belief. For a person to receive healing from God, he must meet three conditions. These may be difficult for someone outside the Church and who has not been through the second birth. One must come to the trueGod, believing that he is petitioning the God of Abraham, Isaac, and Jacob—and the God and Father of the Lord Jesus Christ (Who is also a member of the triune God). He must believe that God is able and willing to heal him, and the belief must be in the heart.

A person may not know if he meets these criteria; but it is always worth asking for healing from God, who is rich in loving kindness, grace, and mercy. No person can speak for another about whether he can meet the criteria; since this information is deep in the heart of a person, the decision is entirely between God and that individual. The Church can guide and provide information, but cannot guarantee a healing from God. There are many things a seeker can do to make it highly likely that God will heal him but these are all natural realm acts and will not allow someone else to know whether the individual is truly making the proper changes in his heart. A person can help another person relate to God but cannot relate to God for him.

Some relevant aspects of God's Character

God's character is performance-oriented with a reward system. All people are equally able to get to the deepest level of reward. Some people have more natural talent and more spiritual gifting; but God, the perfect judge, weighs these things in terms of the work each person performs. He expects greater work from those given more gifting, and these people have a higher level of accountability. The quality of how any individual relates to God is very important to God. If someone does not use his talents, they will be taken away and given to another (Matthew 25:28).

It is very important to understand the role of evil in the creation; and it is very important to understand the roles of infirmity, illness, and injury. God uses illness, infirmity, and injury for correction, training, development of the fruit of the Spirit, for man to see how destructive the negative emotions are, and for him to understand why God wants only those who have the positive emotions in His eternal Kingdom in the future ages. God is very merciful, kind, patient, and loving. Above all He values the truth of His Word in all ages.

The Church in the West is not training members properly to work with God in the ages to come; in this age it is not preparing people to understand the issues related to divine healing.

In 1995 when God healed both authors spontaneously, they tried to understand what had occurred and why. There were only two-authors who made any sense of these issues and who were helpful. None of the several denominations to which we had been exposed ever taught these principles. A review of various statements of belief of major denominations showed a paucity of information with little depth in what was available. God healed Bruce in late 1993, but following this he did not research the issues to any significant extent.

One might ask himself why there is so little teaching in the Church in the West on the subject of divine healing, when healing is so important to God that the Lord Jesus Christ suffered considerably to provide it and since God commands that His children be healed.

Why we have this problem regarding healing in the church doctrines

We are going to illustrate in this example why there is such a problem. When one confines his reasoning to that of the mind which has not been renewed he has to use world system data and methods. He has nothing else as a resource. When one chooses to do this, there will be debates about whether:

a. God still heals,

b. illness and subsequent death are actually good things because then we are with God (*i.e.*, death heals the illness),

c. God uses physicians to heal, and

d. healing is less important than salvation because salvation is the only healing we need.

We have heard many similar statements. When one tries to analyze with surveys and statistics whether there is an issue in the Church regarding healing, he would have to do a large study looking at a lot of data. There would still be debate about the interpretation of that data, the statistical analysis of it, and the methodology of the studies. Such is the way of world system understanding.

Bruce well remembers in 2000 driving home from work listening to a Christian focused radio station carrying a national Bible teacher. This man was denying that healing by God still took place. Bruce, a physician, who well knows the difference between healing provided by a physician and that provided by God and who had experienced several healings of major and minor issues, was sadly not surprised. The example serves to show the failure of the natural mind (either not renewed, or renewed but not mature) to embrace and reason in the supernatural realm. People who deny that healing occurs have hardened their hearts to the miraculous—the individual sin patterns associated with this hardening vary and probably center mostly on not renewing the mind and on not taking thoughts captive. A major Biblical example of the same is found in Mark 8:15-21. These apostles had lived in the presence of God for many months but had never renewed their minds. It is so important for the Church to teach taking thoughts captive, renewal of the mind, purification of the heart, and praise and worship of God. Without obediently performing these commandments of God, one can never get beyond the natural realm to live and function in the spiritual realm.

If one has a renewed mind and is taking his thoughts captive, he learns how to communicate with God; and then he works with God to develop his spiritual senses. If he does not develop these, he cannot live in the spiritual realm. After learning to communicate with God, one can confidently ask God any question he wishes. We have asked God to choose what make and color car we should purchase, and He is always pleased to advise a person. One is much more likely to get a car that will be relatively issue-free. God is always pleased to answer questions about the creation and Himself. God will not answer a question from a doubleminded man (James 1:5-8).

The spiritual realm answer to the above question

When one has a renewed mind and is used to understanding and operating in the spiritual realm, he will turn to God first to ask for spiritual realm wisdom, understanding, and knowledge whenever there is an issue. God always provides an answer in a way which gives a complete understanding and which will stand through the ages.

In 1998 a church meeting of eight area churches in Lancaster, Pennsylvania was called to pray to God to break a harsh drought. Alta Ada asked Bruce, who was always reticent in those days to socialize more than he had to if they would attend. He said that he did not think it necessary and that we could join in prayer without going to the meeting. The morning of the prayer meeting while Bruce was driving to work the Holy Spirit said to him: "If you are going to live in the community, you might at least go and pray for it." We do not recall who was more surprised that they were going to the meeting—Bruce or Alta Ada. At that meeting the Lord spoke to Bruce and said that He was going to break the drought; but He added that the churches are weak and that God wanted him to teach His people about how to be led by the Spirit of God.

When God makes a statement like that, one does not need surveys or statistics to know that the churches in the West are weak. Bruce had been preparing for this ministry since he first knew that God wanted him to teach people how to be led by His Spirit within a few weeks of receiving the second birth.

Some health care questions we have asked of God include:

Why are we are seeing so few healings in the church in the west?

One night driving home from work in about 2006 Bruce was talking to God about why we see so few people in the churches healed. God did not dispute the question and answered that it is because people want faith to be healed but they do not want faith in God (His Character). Thus, a difficult question in the natural realm about healing is resolved in a five minute discussion with God. The bottom line is that people do not want to get to know God; but they would like to be healed by Him. God also affirmed the reason for fewer healings and the correction for the problem.

How do you feel about the United States health care system?

Around 1996 Bruce asked God about His thoughts on the United States health care system. Within two to three minutes the Lord answered the question, as He frequently does, with Scripture. He quoted this Scripture:

Proverbs 20:10

[10] Divers weights, *and* divers measures, both of them *are* alike abomination to the LORD.

Interestingly, God did not quote it verbatim but said: "False weights, poor measure; an abomination."

This does not mean there is no good thing in the United States health care system, and it does not mean that all people working in it are doing a poor job. The statement stands as it is. God was saying that there was not the value in it for the population. This does not indicate in any way that God was advocating a particular change or a particular system. We have never asked these questions of God. We suspect that, if we did, the answer would be to bring back the church in the community to being the salt and light that God wants it to be; then the burden of illness in the United States would fall dramatically.

Bruce was really struggling about writing this book early in the summer of 2017 while Alta Ada was having a lot of health issues. In discussing his concern with God, Bruce received this answer. "Don't you have faith to write the book?" God frequently is quite brief in his answers but they go straight to the point. Fear was behind the concern about writing the book; as this became apparent Bruce started again on the book.

We have used more personal anecdotes in this chapter and throughout the book on the advice and encouragement of God speaking through our close friend, Bishop Willie L. Cage of Hammond, Louisiana. We like to use Scripture to tell the story and arrange the text about the Scriptures in the books we write. This brings the reader to the living Word of God.

The reason for these anecdotes above is to highlight the greatest cause of weakness in the Church in the West. The reason is that, in general, the Church has lost its connection with its head, the Lord Jesus Christ. This is a general statement and in no way reflects on every single church congregation.

We will now look at the issues in the church in the West which have led to the declining numbers of attendees, loss of societal influence, and contempt from many outside the church. After this we will look at solutions which God is suggesting. One can diagnose a pervasive spiritual illness in the church because it is failing to perform adequately the many works God has given it. Spiritual illnesses always have a natural realm outworking. These are the natural realm symptoms that we see and which result from the spiritual problems.

Signs in the Natural Realm in the United States that show weakening of the church

There are several organizations which do societal surveys looking at religious behavior and beliefs. One can readily access these survey results. They show the following results.

There is a decline in numbers of people going to a church.

There is steeper decline in younger people going to a church.

A quite small number of church attendees hold the Bible to be without error

There is a decline of people who identify with the church who believe the Biblical creation account.

There is a decrease in the perception that God is Holy and that He will punish all sin, and thus a decrease in believing that there is only one way to Heaven and that through the salvation offered by the Lord Jesus Christ.

Many people associated with the church now believe that God accepts the worship of all religions, that one's good works will get them a place in heaven, that science has disproved the Biblical account in several areas, and that the Bible is not purely the written word of God. There are many similar surveys all of which show the same trends.

We have to look at the spiritual problems which have led to this watering down of the truth in Western societies. God reveals to man in His interactions with individuals and in His foundational setting Scriptures recorded in the Bible a truth which is very different from the generally-held perceptions, reviewed above, among those who attend a church. Unless the spiritual problems in the Church are corrected, there is no way the natural-realm symptoms from them will be corrected. We will look at spiritual realm symptoms in the Church, and then we will look at the spiritual illnesses behind these symptoms.

The Spiritual Symptoms

All of these spiritual symptoms result from a very simple issue—that there is a great loss of the experiential knowledge of the character of God in the Church at both the leadership and the individual levels. This, in turn, results from a loss of spiritual hearing and vision which stems from a failure of those in the Church to understand how to mature in their spirit man. When people do not experience a deepening and broadening relationship with God, then they will allow their natural-realm thinking to explain spiritual realm matters. All too often, their natural-realm thinking is strongly mixed with world system thoughts and philosophies. These thoughts and philosophies can be laid at the feet of the powers of darkness. Following are some of the results:

1. There is **little unity in the spirit** between large parts of the professing members of the Church. This lack of unity is not just in the natural realm, where it could be due

just to differences in administration in the local churches. Rather, lack of unity is in the spiritual realm. Lack of unity in the spirit is strongly related to a lack of spiritual maturity; and as a result of this immaturity there is little understanding of the character of God.

2. There is a major **loss of knowledge of the character of God** in the Church which leads to large-scale unbelief in the people of God. There is a significant loss of the ability to communicate back and forth with God in both Church leadership and in Church members.

3. There is rising **disregard for the supernatural realm of God** in most Western societies that is evidenced in many behavior patterns. These areas include family values, esteem for life, esteem for His Word, and separation from the world system.

4. **The Church tries to influence through secular means instead of through spiritual power.** This is a mistaken way of addressing the world's problems. God does not stop people outside His own family from self-destructing behavior. He even facilitates it when he has made sure that an individual will not turn to Him in repentance for behavior which He abhors. God has the power to feed all of the hungry, clothe all of the poor, and give everyone a fine dwelling. There is nothing wrong with performing these ministries; and indeed they are needed—feeding the poor, clothing people, and providing shelter. The problem is there is no spiritual foundation. One can give a person a fish, but it is better to give him the means of fishing. Just so, one can give natural-realm assistance; but it has to be linked strongly to demonstrations of spiritual power. What would impress a person more—giving him a piece of bread or multiplying five loaves to feed thousands?

Frequently, the church tries to legislate morality through political and legal processes. There is nothing wrong with this, but it would be more effective to be able to bring God's character to a person. A person caught in a sin pattern might feel unclean and thus be motivated to change.

5. **There is little understanding of what God's agenda for the creation is.** Since His agenda is very different from the agendas of men before their second birth and even after it, this results in a lack of prayer for God's causes and a weakening of the power in the Church.

6. **There is a marked decline in supernatural functioning in the Church in the West.**

7. **The Church is not focusing on Serving God.** Instead, it focuses on fixing the world as its mission; and that is not what God has called it to do. The primary focus of the Church should be to teach every member to come into a relationship with God and to do what He utters to them. He has to coordinate all of the activities of all of His people. We do not have the knowledge and understanding of how to do that. The Church, when it focuses on the problems of the world, is essentially in a situation of elevating the creation above the Creator. This is similar to what many unbelieving people do.

All of these symptoms are related to spiritual illness in the Church. These spiritual illnesses are robbing the Church of its ability to carry out the many things that God has wants it to do. We will now look at the root disease which has been unleashed in the Church, and then we can consider the secondary illnesses that stem from that. Then we can examine the solutions that God suggests. God showed Bruce the problems and the solutions early in 2017.

The Church in the West is weak in the spiritual realm; as a result, it is weak in the natural realm. One must adjust his thinking considerably if he is to understand these points. Some (perhaps most) can be spiritually discerned only; while these ideas may fairly self-evident, the concept is going to take some spiritual growth for full revelation.

1 Corinthians 2:14–15

[14] But the natural man receiveth not the things of the Spirit of God: for they are foolishness unto him: neither can he know *them*, because they are spiritually discerned. [15] But he that is spiritual judgeth all things, yet he himself is judged of no man.

Many people reading the Scripture above will think that they understand it. The Scripture itself states that this is impossible. One has to decide whether he believes his own mind or the Word of God. This is perhaps the key problem in the spiritual realm. Men these days think, based on their behavior, that they know more than God knows; and yet He has told men that His thoughts and His ways are higher than those of men. As one grows in the spiritual realm, he will gradually come to understand what this Scripture is saying. It cannot be understood without spiritual maturity.

Implications for Church Leadership of this decline in power in both the natural and spiritual realms

When people in leadership fail to respond to major issues that concern God about the spiritual condition and spiritual health of His people, then they are confusing to whom they are called to minister to and to whom their allegiance belongs. They may face future wrath from God for failing to respond to these issues. Both leaders and all members of the Church need to repent for the current spiritual climate in the West. This climate reflects a loss of the saltiness of the Church. The function of the Church is to be salt and light to a society; and when it fails to perform this role, then there is a great loss for society. All individuals in the Church need to repent for their spiritual immaturity. This spiritual immaturity is pervasive and limits success in carrying out God's plans, which include taking back the works of the devil. Our wars are never against people. In recent times the Church has tried to respond to the problems with carnal weapons, such as using political solutions for moral problems, instead of using spiritual power. Political weapons will never work well, as they are against people.

God is merciful and gracious. Even now, if leadership in the Church would work together toward correcting the gross spiritual immaturity, then God would be like the father of the prodigal son. He would come running to meet us. We need to understand God and His ways.

The battle for the souls of men and the Spirit of False Knowledge

One has to look at the historical battles for the souls of men between God and the evil spirits—including the devil, Satan. Throughout history Satan has tried to stop God's plans for mankind and His plans for the creation (Revelation 12:3-9). Satan has never been able to succeed, although he can cause and has caused much suffering and misery for many people. However, he was defeated at the cross by the Lord Jesus Christ. Since this defeat more than 2,000 years ago the devil has concentrated on weakening the quality of the spirits of men in the Church; in addition, he has tried to limit the quantity of God's inheritance for eternity by many means. Currently he uses abortion, drugs, alcohol, violent crime, "accidental injuries," and war. At the individual level he works to prevent a person, experiencing the second birth by all of the considerable forces at his disposal. If a person does go through the second birth, then Satan's plan is to prevent maturing of the new soul and spirit and thereby to sideline the new creation from being useful to God.

One should note that whenever man is able to invent something to get God's Words before people, such as the printing press, the devil will pervert the good that these inventions can bring. The same sequence is observed in the information age where men, formed in the image of God and having innate creative abilities, have been able to develop all of the current electronics and software which so enhance all of our work abilities. Initially, all were developed for the serving of mankind. Subsequently, evil spirits have influenced some men to use these tools for crime, exploitation of immoral purposes, and manipulation of other people.

The Enlightenment

Perhaps the devil's greatest attack on God through mankind began between 1650 and 1700 with the Age of the Enlightenment (also known as the Age of Reason). A powerful evil spiritual being came against God in this movement and since has recruited beneath it many other layers of spiritual powers who continue to spawn further false wisdom, false understanding, and false knowledge into a foundation for the world system as it currently functions.

In this period there was a strong emphasis on scientific method and reductionism, which describes everything as being a part of the individual components. A major problem with reductionism is that it leaves out spiritual realm interactions because it concentrates on just the natural realm. At the same time there arose a strong attack on the prior religious orthodoxy.

Resulting philosophies which have come from this spirit of false wisdom, false understanding, and false knowledge include Darwinism (evolution), which is still increasing in influence and which is directly opposed to God's creation account. This, in turn, has led to the evils of Nazism with supremacy of the species. Many of the major philosophies have come from this spirit of false wisdom, understanding, and knowledge (Isaiah 11:2). High level powers of evil operate these thought systems against mankind.

The Church has failed to recognize fully the evil of the spirit of knowledge which acts through the natural realm and which attempts to block all access to and knowledge of the spiritual realm. There has never been any successfully organized defense by the Church against this very high level evil spirit.

The Church is now in a situation in which even those who recognize that there is a problem tend to discuss it in the very terms of the enemy (using natural-realm reasoning) and try to address it through natural counter-knowledge. This spirit tries to suppress knowledge of and access to the power of God operating through the natural realm. It tries to counter the miraculous acts of God by reason and scientific explanations.

Outcomes of the work of this spirit of false knowledge and its network of subservient spirits

We will look at several outcomes from the attack by this spirit of false wisdom, understanding, and knowledge that are issues which continue to cause the current poor spiritual health in the Church in the West. This spirit of false knowledge (1 Corinthians 3:18-20) has robbed the Church of its connection to the spiritual head, the Lord Jesus Christ; and as a result the body decides on actions independently of its head. In addition, the body has lost a lot of the knowledge of the Head and understands His character poorly. The Church also has lost the power that it would have if it were in close fellowship to the Lord God. It is also failing to grow in spiritual power and maturity because the attention and focus are on operating in the natural realm. Indeed, there is little understanding of the two realms and how they are related and how they interact. An example of this confusion is that few understand that the body of flesh is the earthly Temple of God (1 Corinthians 3:16-17). The statement is self-evident, but the issues behind it are poorly understood. The seven spiritual symptoms listed above are the result of the work of this spirit and the work of the hierarchy of lower-level spirits under its direction.

The Secularization of the West

This spirit of false knowledge and the hierarchy of evil under it have secularized the Western countries and have done this through advancing sciences and seductive philosophies centered about evolution. This spirit has challenged some of the truths of the revelation of God; His Church has not defended these truths well. This spirit has been able to entrench itself through science and has dazzled men by the power that has been discovered in fossil fuels and in the atomic fuels. The Information Age has also subverted people into spending much more of their time on entertainment. What it has done effectively is to blind people to the truth of the forest in which they live by captivating them with the knowledge of the trees so that they never look again at the forest. This spirit of false knowledge has elevated humanism in all its forms from the philosophy of humanism to the demonstration of man's ability to control much of his environment through technology, including;modern medical advances.

This spirit has captured the education systems of Western countries; since most children are exposed to education systems, those who ultimately go through the second birth have to undo much learning, believing, and attitudes.

This spirit has made people labor in learning and has yoked them to being busy perpetually. People tend to know a lot of trivia, but few are able to contemplate the spiritual issues of the environment in which they live. They are kept in the woods and never see the forest and what is beyond it.

The same spirit has increased entertainment options which allow people to stay busy when not working. When one is being entertained, he is not pondering and meditating about substantial issues—which is exactly what these evil spirits desire and plan.

The attack on the Genesis creation account

This spirit has also been able to attack the accuracy of the Scriptures through such issues as the age of the universe. The contention is that scientists have "proven" the earth to be older than the creation account. Since science and all of the intellect behind it seem very powerful, even the Church has not been able to defend adequately in the public mind. Since theologians are usually not scientists in this age of educational specialization, the voices of scientists backing creation (there are many who do) have been drowned out in the public forum. We, the authors, think that, while the work of these scientists is good, they have not been able to attack the root of this spirit in the spiritual realm and have confined most of their work to countering natural-realm arguments with natural realm findings. The engagement has to be spirit against spirit, not natural-realm understanding versus natural-realm understanding. Most natural understanding poorly represents the truth of the spiritual realm and is almost entirely false due to the vanity to which the creation is subject. The creation is in death throes and basically is like a decomposing body with *rigor mortis*. It does not represent spiritual life except where God gives miracles and where people carry a strong measure of the Spirit of Life.

Attacks on the miracles

The spirit of false knowledge has leveraged this attack against creation truth into attacks on the miracles by supplying natural explanations. The human sciences have been laced with false knowledge. In the sciences in which pure observational work is done (*e.g.*, mathematics) the outcomes are closer to true knowledge. Scientists cannot explain the miracles in natural-realm terms. When a scientist tries to interpret the past and the future, he is uses false knowledge because there is no spiritual-realm component to the research. There is no understanding that the dying and moribund nature of the creation is all that he sees in the natural realm. This state of death affects all measurements, which project both backward and forward and confuses any scientific inferences even approximating truth. When God develops one's spiritual vision, he can see the abundant life that is present in the spiritual realm. It is only as God opens up a person's spiritual senses as he matures that he can start to reason with spiritual-realm observations. Bruce will never forget the opening of his eyes to see a mantle of shimmering evil layered over all of the picturesque geography of the area in which he lives.

The heavy erosion of the beliefs in spiritual-realm understanding coming from reductionism, coupled with observational sciences, has dealt a heavy blow to the learning of spiritual-realm knowledge. People in the Church have absorbed these natural realm based philosophies; as a result, their hearts have hardened to consideration of the miraculous—which still frequently occurs. We looked earlier at the issue of a hardened heart. The exposure of young people to the secular educational systems in the West have made many who have been through the second birth very hardened to the full truth of the creation account in Genesis and to the truth of the miracles. A person can change this only by coming to know God personally. After going through the second birth, the new spiritual babe does not know God well. Unless he is trained to know and to communicate with God he never will know much more than *facts* about God. Spiritual infants who are not growing cannot have the power of God. Yes, someone might be able to perform a healing because of a spiritual gift; but this is a very limited occurrence which will seem almost a random act and therefore will show little of the character of God.

We will now look at some of the thoughts that God has given Bruce as he pondered the current situation. There are some major categories which we will examine under the heading of the pervasive secularism in the Church. We have made some of these points previously, but we will repeat them due to the nature of these revelations. These are all general observations and might not apply to some individual congregations.

Current Church Leadership Issues

The Church has lost the connection with the Head, and this loss results in church leadership making policy and giving direction under the veneer of praying about it; but it rarely listens for God to direct. There are various types of governance; but churches usually choose people to be on boards based on their secular skills and not on faithfulness to and intimacy with God. Churches use secular models for the training and selection of pastors and lay leaders. There is usually only a small modicum of spiritual insight.

As a result, we have a clear division between ministry and members. College-/and/or seminary-educated people now lead most ministry. They have taken academic programs, but some may never have had a true calling from God. There is no incentive to train the members—indeed, that could spell competition. There are no, or few, seminary programs which focus on the supernatural realm. Seminary instructors have learned how to become "indispensable" to the Church, and thus justify their own continuance. They are very unlikely to focus on any idea that God should select the students; although they may pray over lists. The whole model is not too far from that of the Pharisees' models.

The background of students admitted to seminary tends to omit or diminish the science backgrounds; thus the Church is not keeping up with the natural-realm revelation of God's creation and hence is not able to counter it with spiritual-realm truth about the true mechanisms in the creation. This has been an ongoing weakness in the Church.

Church has become entertainment-oriented to fill the pews, fill the "coffers," and maintain the buildings. There is a pressure on leadership from the Boards to keep the buildings and physical plant working. Oftentimes, financial decisions are the ones that lead the people to seek God for direction; but since many hardened hearts are present, hearing God is not easy.

The Church has not been equipping the members properly.

We feel that one reason for this is considerably related to the issue that much of the Church ignores a large and vitally important part of Scripture. This part is the need for the Church to equip those who have been through the second birth for service in God's Kingdom. A second reason is that the churches are omitting Scriptures dealing with the process for equipping. Books and articles about how to equip the Church people tend to be focus on what the end result should be and to omit the mechanics for achieving this end result. Therefore, they do not solve the problem. People know there is an issue, but they seem to have little thought about how to solve it. The situation is one that seems to have come about as the Church, in general, has gradually dipped into a very pervasive and seductive form of secularism. This results in people's going through an experience they call the second birth but never growing into spiritual maturity. Many who think that they have received the second birth actually may not have. Demons are very well able to induce fleshly emotion and excitement and thus confuse people. Secularism tends to grow when spiritual-realm vision fades.

In using this term *spiritual vision*, we are not talking about prophecy in the sense of a person's gaining a word from a prophet for encouragement at a service. We are talking about a prophetic insight from the Lord God for His Church in the West. At this time there is a great level of secularization in the Churches in the Western nations. This may not be readily apparent to the individual worshiping in a local church that gives him good support, but nonetheless it is strongly present organizationally; and we will discuss some of the causes. If one wishes to model the Church on the New Testament, Watchman Nee's book *The Normal Christian Church Life* would be very helpful.

Some causes for the pervasive secularism in the Church in the West and for the current problems in the Church in the West

We are going to list some issues for the Church and some causes of secularism. We will then make some suggestions about strategies for overcoming the problems. God gave these revelations to Bruce in meditations at night. These revelations are not additions to God's Word but personal enlightenment on the content from the Holy Spirit.

1. When one goes through the second birth, he is an infant in the spiritual realm. At the second birth one is born into an entirely new realm with rules of operation that are very different from rules in the natural realm. Unless the person is trained by God, Himself (assisted by spiritually mature programs and Church leaders), then that person never

develops spiritual senses. The spiritual realm means nothing to him, and so he continues to operate in the natural realm. Hebrews 5:11-14 describes this lack of development. It results in what the Apostle Paul would label a "carnal believer." Such people can be very little different in their thinking and understanding of the spiritual realm in comparison from those who have never been through the second birth.

2. There is a lack of spiritually mature leadership in many local churches (not all). The selection of candidates and the training for the ministry have been performed in a secularized manner, so that a trained mind becomes a substitute for a maturing spirit. If people even think about spiritual maturity, they frequently substitute academic knowledge for it. We need to remember clearly that the mind and the spirit of a person are two very different parts of the soul. Development of the intellect does not parallel spiritual maturity. Bruce had a patient who, due to limited natural-realm mental abilities, needed custodial care at age 18. This man was seeing light and dark angels and was committed to the Lord God. His spiritual-realm vision was more advanced than many other people that Bruce has met. Of course, if one is to teach and inspire others in his sphere, he must be talented in the pertinent natural realm issues and be able to teach the ideas. An example of needing the natural-realm knowledge is of Daniel and his friends (Daniel 1:4).

3. Many people in church leadership understand the concept of spirit very poorly; thus, they rarely discuss it with or teach it to the lay members. Spirit is the very nature of God, who is spirit. Not to discuss and understand *spirit* puts the Church into a very unwise place with God. One cannot understand how to communicate properly with God without understanding the Biblical revelation of *spirit*. Not understanding this need does not prevent the

relationship, but it slows down the development of the relationship and impairs the depth of it. God states the following:

John 4:23–24

[23] But the hour cometh, and now is, when the true worshippers shall worship the Father in spirit and in truth: for the Father seeketh such to worship him. [24] God *is* a Spirit: and they that worship him must worship *him* in spirit and in truth.

It is not possible to attain this ideal without understanding the issues of spirit and of truth. One must be able to discern reliably the movement of his spirit as distinct from that of his flesh and mind. This discernment comes with practice. In worship one must make sure that it is his spirit which is initiating and maintaining the worship, not his flesh. If the mind is renewed, then it can work with the spirit to worship God. People generally neglect the issue of truth in this passage. God is the source of true wisdom, true understanding, and true knowledge. One must worship Him within the framework of His truth (not wisdom of the world system). Therefore, we cannot worship Him using the world's wisdom, understanding, and knowledge—for none of that is truth. God's understanding of truth is much higher than what natural man would deem truth. Truth exists primarily in the spiritual realm and not in the natural realm. Only the things of God are truth; but beyond this the carefully-made observations in the natural realm sometime approximate truth, but nothing pertaining to the world system has truth in it. God speaks to us in natural circumstances, but we then have to discuss the issues about the circumstances with Him to discern His intent for us. The Church and the people of the Church have to live within the world system (as with Daniel and his friends) and operate in it for the work of God in redemption; but we need to keep the overall perspective of being in the world but not of it (1 John 2:15).

4. The churches for the most part have divided members into lay and professional categories, which is not what the Apostle Paul discussed in Ephesians 4:10-13. There should be no division since all saints are to be equipped. Furthermore, all teachers and all trainees should aspire to the same endpoint of becoming a perfect man. This is clearly not occurring in many local churches.

Ephesians 4:10–13

[10] He that descended is the same also that ascended up far above all heavens, that he might fill all things.) [11] And he gave some, apostles; and some, prophets; and some, evangelists; and some, pastors and teachers; [12] For the perfecting of the saints, for the work of the ministry, for the edifying of the body of Christ: [13] Till we all come in the unity of the faith, and of the knowledge of the Son of God, unto a perfect man, unto the measure of the stature of the fulness of Christ.

The saints are not being perfected. All church members need to be perfected unto the stature of the Lord Jesus in His power and character. This is what God expects; He demands much of those in leadership and will hold people accountable for failing in this requirement. We do not come to unity of the faith because we do not see God very well, due to poorly developed spiritual senses and a poorly-developed relationship with God. When a person is not able to use spiritual senses, he will "fill in the blanks," so to speak, with world system false understanding. Most lay members do not seem to be aware of the need for spiritual growth. They see God to the depth of their own involvement with Him, which is quite variable.

5. The enormous demands on Church members from the

world system facilitate secularization of the church. This wears down faith and belief and weakens the individual members. We discuss this below.

Romans 12:2

² And be not conformed to this world: but be ye transformed by the renewing of your mind, that ye may prove what *is* that good, and acceptable, and perfect, will of God.

God is telling us (through the Apostle Paul) that the usual situation in the world system setting is that people of the Church are conformed to it. Therefore, we have to seek His solution to prevent this usual outcome. People are going to be conformed to the things to which they devote their time and resources. The Scriptures teach that "where your treasure is will be where your heart (core of your being) is." We may think and wish that our treasure is elsewhere; but that is counter to Scripture, and Scripture is truth because God is truth.

Secularization in our work

God has given us the solution. In our core we must always seek God, and then we will see His hand in all situations including world system situations. This occurs by the renewing of the spirit of the mind. If we devote our time to the world system, we will be part of it. However, if we constantly are taking our thoughts captive and looking to see what God is doing in every circumstance (1 Thessalonians 5:17-18), then He will be with us in our secular work and will enable us to be more effective and efficient in it. Daniel (Daniel 1:4) and his friends were given wisdom in the ways of the world system, and yet Daniel and his friends kept their primary focus on God. Sometimes this brings one into confrontation with the system, as it did Daniel's friends, but at other times it sways the ruler, as it did later in Daniel's case. This is part of the renewing of the mind. God will give us skill in the world system ways to do His work, if we keep our focus on Him first.

Titus 2:12

[12] Teaching us that, denying ungodliness and worldly lusts, we should live soberly, righteously, and godly, in this present world;

Here God tells us how we are to live in a secularized world system. We see that ungodliness is not the same as lust.

2 Timothy 2:16

[16] But shun profane *and* vain babblings: for they will increase unto more ungodliness.

Secularization in worship

Vain is "empty," and *profane* is "secular." Vain babblings include such things as the mantra type of repetitive singing or speaking repetitive phrases. God is highly intelligent and expects us to be lucid in our communications with Him. He does not expect polished language skills. He takes us as we are and expects us to talk with Him in a manner similar to what we would use with a revered and close friend. We would not chant repetitive phrases to a friend, although we might plead and repeat ourselves a few times. The Scriptures ask us to be persistent but frown on vain repetition.

There has been much secularization in the music in the Church and in the worship service format. Some churches actually do marketing surveys and use marketing technology (this is world system) to reach people. When the root of anything is unholy (secular), the fruit will never be holy (Romans 11:16-17).

6. As a result of secularization and the resulting lack of spiri-

tual maturity there is not much progression in people after the second birth beyond the one experience with God at the time of the second birth. People have to progress in knowing God personally, similar to progressing in getting to know a friend (time and commitment). There are some who have occasional interactions with God and fewer who have had a lot of interactions with Him; but even then people try to understand God by using what is called world system (false knowledge in God's view) knowledge to try to explain spiritual knowledge. This just does not work. A typical example is when a Church sends out a survey to see how members are aligned with respect to an issue. The church will then make some change in the Church operations based on the survey. The correct way is to seek God's solutions in prayerful intercession; but the fact that this is not the method shows the lack of closeness the people have with God. To whom does the Church belong? It is God's, and it does not belong to the people who attend. Secularization causes a faulty concept (as revealed by the way it transacts business) of whom the local church body belongs to.

God wants us to pray without ceasing (1 Thessalonians 5:17). Praying without ceasing is being in a state in our heart in which we stay in God's presence. We know we are in His presence when our spirit stays filled with peace and joy and when we are righteous (Romans 14:17). In this situation our spirit is sensitive to the slightest movement of His Spirit; we are waiting on Him to do His bidding. When the people of the Church are not trained in how to do this, secularization results and worsens as the lack of prayer increases. People grow in spiritual strength when they wait on God and turn things over to His decision making. We would never expect natural infants to make policy decisions for a company; similarly, we should not ask spiritual infants to make decisions (through surveys) for God.

Some will say that by doing something like a survey, people feel included. They may feel more included in a humanistic worldly club into which the church in the West is moving rapidly; but they will not feel more included in the plans of God.

7. A lot of so-called praise music consists of repetitions; this is of the world. It is another area in which the secularized Church lacks spiritual discernment. We are even aware of some local churches allowing such practices as yoga. They use the excuse that it is "just exercise." However, the root is unholy, since the source is in Eastern religions. The fruit will also be unholy (this is obvious with spiritual discernment). In the natural realm yoga may be just a different type of exercise; and so it is to the natural-realm mind. In the spiritual realm we can see the demonic origins and control. God does not own yoga; it is a plant of the evil spirits. Freemasonry at lower levels may appear innocent, but at the higher levels it quickly shows itself to be the worshiping of demons, especially Satan. Higher levels of yoga are similar; and while not all people go into these deeper levels, there is still harm to the spirit which becomes unclean before God and subject to His cursing. God's people must be Holy and separated from the world system—especially from demonic activities and worship.

If such issues were just natural-realm issues then such entities as yoga would be all right. All issues involve both the natural and spiritual realm, and it takes developed spiritual discernment to see why something that looks all right in the natural realm can be quite evil (Hebrews 5:12-14). The Scriptures are quite clear about the fruit being related to the root. This and other situations show a lack of spiritual discernment among the leadership of local bodies which permit such things. Natural discernment will always be at enmity with the Spirit of God. Discernment is a product of spiritual growth (Hebrews 5:11-14). The lack of it shows the general weakness of spiritual growth and strength in local church bodies.

8. Many pastors and leaders (also a large number of people in the Church) fear man more than God, at least in some circumstances. This fear influences much of the local church management. In some geographic areas the state provides a form of support to the church with tax exemptions for donations. Once a church accepts these benefits, it can be quite dependent on them; and there are rules that stop some freedom of speech which comes with these benefits. The problem is that since a lot of social issues are politicized, pastors are compromised from speaking forthrightly on God's principles regarding such issues.

The result of fearing man more than God plays out in many issues, other than directly finance related; but even then at the root of most of these issues there may be a financial concern. The whole concept is not healthy for the church. God set up one form of governance for the state and a different form of governance for the Church. Concern about God's provision in the matter of finances probably is the underlying cause for fearing man above fearing God. God promises to provide always for one's needs. He will not underwrite programs that are secular, since we do not need them. If a church is having financial issues it should examine what it is doing that is not pleasing to God.

We have quoted Scripture elsewhere recounting where the Lord Jesus paid tribute money (taxes) for Peter and Himself in order not to offend the authorities. This would seem to be the principle: instead of operating on the tax-free margin it might be wise for local church bodies to consider operating on a lower revenue stream and donating extra income to a worthwhile cause. Churches should consider changing this dependence on tax-free revenue.

In decisions, both related to and unrelated to finances, local church leadership really should be seeking what God wants in all decisions—the members are His sheep. The Church collectively works only to the extent that the Lord Jesus is both the titular head and the operating and functional head. If He is replaced from His role in any area, that area becomes secularized.

9. Believing God is a major issue for individuals and for the local church. It is as important as having faith in God. Faith comes from knowing one has heard God's answer to a prayer. Belief is dependent on knowing God's character. Both faith and belief are very important. Faith involves spiritual hearing. Belief involves knowing God personally in the heart, and this is entirely different from believing with the mind. When one believes something in his heart, he acts on information pertinent to it. Until one believes something in the heart, he is building just a mental structure that is like the house built on sand. It will not stand when trouble comes. The spiritual strength of an individual is directly related to his experiential knowledge of God's character and of His abilities. He gains this knowledge through many experiences—with his mind renewed, his heart purified, and his spiritual senses operating. We need to focus in the Church on making sure people understand how to believe in the heart and how to work with God to tear down old structures and to let Him build new structures.

10. Decision making is frequently highly secularized. It is an area which needs much strengthening. In this respect the closeness of a decision to God's perfect will is dependent on the ability of the individual decision makers to understand how to discern God's will. Church teaching needs to address being led by God in personal decision making. It is only through being led by God in decsion making that an individual can purify his heart. At the foundation of

purifying his heart is the need to be renewed in the spirit of his mind and to take all of his thoughts captive for the Lord Jesus Christ. 2 Corinthians 10:5 commands the following:

1. Cast down imaginations that elevate the self, the world system, and the creation itself. They frequently dictate our purchasing and our socializing.

2. Cast down anything that is false wisdom, understanding, and knowledge; hold God's knowledge as the goal of all understanding and wisdom.

3. Examine even the smallest and seemingly trivial thoughts for the motive and for the individual being honored. Over time one will see patterns, and this will become automatic. It would help to practice it for an hour daily.

11. Another important issue is that the infiltration of secular thinking into the Church in the West leads it to provide secular solutions to the needs of communities. This secularization is related to the falling away of the knowledge of God—His Character, His power; and His ways. When this fades, then faith in God is lost. God has designed man in such a way that he needs to put his faith in something (Micah 4:5). Without faith in God, which can come only through a relationship of bilateral communication, man turns to the early secularized training and learning he received through the education system; thereby believing in the creature rather than the Creator for decision making. When one is thinking primarily about secular issues and is seeking secular solutions,his mind has not been renewed in the way God requests; and thus he functions primarily in the natural realm. This makes him spiritually blind to the extent he does this. He may see some spiritual truth, but not nearly as much as he should (1 Corinthians 2:14-15 below). Secular thinking influences the ability to

perceive truth. This is probably no more apparent than in the proclivity to use the results of statistical studies for decision making, without fully understanding their limitations. In many minds they offer proof of cause and effect; of course, this is untrue.

The use of secular thought and thinking leads to difficulty for several reasons in identifying truth. This secularization of the thoughts and thinking of people in the local churches, even after they have been through the second birth, leads to very unwise decisions. This, in turn, leads to a very false image of God being presented to the community by the church. it distorts His character and His abilities; and He is frequently presented as someone who is not involved in the affairs of His people, *i.e.*, a distant and removed deity. This book is our attempt to encourage people to start to understand the character and the abilities of our only true and very much living and involved God. His ownership of the creation and where He is going with it are not getting into our communities. This will lead to many lost souls.

12. Faith, Hope, Love, and Belief

We dealt with these issues in Chapter 7. Faith and belief are two closely-related and very important spiritual attributes in each individual who has been through the second birth. To be successful in spiritual battles, one needs understanding and development of both faith and belief. In addition, our ability to give love to God and our ability to receive it from Him are critical to obtaining spiritual strength and power.

The secular community sees faith as trust, and perhaps most people in the Church would see it in the same way. People assume that they understand belief. Both faith and belief have a natural and a spiritual realm component. Unfortunately, the spiritual-realm structures of both faith and belief are not well understood. Belief is so important for spiritual battles. We will review some of the Scriptures which we looked at in Chapter 7.

A foundational Scripture that places faith in the spiritual realm instead of just in the natural realm is the following:

Romans 10:17

[17] So then faith *cometh* by hearing, and hearing by the word of God.

The Greek word for *word* is *rhema*, which is the continued utterances of God to individuals. Therefore, without hearing God and His directions for any particular decision one cannot have faith in that issue; a vague overall belief in God and that He will support conclusions drawn from His written Word are all that are left. He might do this; but there is not much power in this, and one obtains the "good" will of God instead of the "perfect" will of God (Romans 12:2). Therefore, to be effective for God, we must be able to converse reliably with Him. It is no use thinking that perhaps we heard Him. This really is a form of unbelief. Below is a critical Scripture for belief.

Mark 11:23–24

[23] For verily I say unto you, That whosoever shall say unto this mountain, Be thou removed, and be thou cast into the sea; and shall not doubt in his heart, but shall believe that those things which he saith shall come to pass; he shall have whatsoever he saith. [24] Therefore I say unto you, What things soever ye desire, when ye pray, believe that ye receive *them*, and ye shall have *them*.

The issues are that one shall not doubt in His heart and that he must believe that his request will come to pass—with no room for doubt. To be able to fulfill these conditions, one must have both the right spiritual structures built in his heart and spiritual warfare expertise. This will enable one to defend attacks on belief from a spirit of doubt. God has to train one to acquire expertise in spiritual warfare. He can choose his weapons from passages in God's Word. God will equip each of His children according to individual experiences He has given him. The Scripture 2 Timothy 2:13 gives one of the strongest weapons we have in God's Word, the fact that God will defend the truth in His Word; but not many know how to use it. No one can succeed in spiritual warfare unless God has trained him and is with him.

2 Timothy 2:13

[13] If we believe not, *yet* he abideth faithful: he cannot deny himself.

This Scripture tells us that God will always maintain his activities consistent with His revelations in the Scriptures. This gives structure to both the spiritual and natural realms which will transcend time. His Word is a major structural element in the spiritual and natural realms. In a spiritual battle with an evil spirit that spirit is constrained by God's Word. We can take advantage of that to successfully pray against that spirit. God will have to defend His Word.

If we do not use the spiritual weapons of Ephesians 6 to fight battles but instead use secularized philosophies and understandings, then we will be unlikely to be successful in spiritual warfare. If we use secular arguments and reasoning, we will be fighting in the devil's own princedom. Fighting in the spiritual realm and seeing the issues in that realm are what is required to bring the victory against the devil (Colossians 2:5).

13. Fighting Battles

God instructs the people of the Church to use the whole armor that He supplies. He specifically defined the enemy as evil spirits and not men. In this area of battling spiritual foes the Church seems generally to use natural-realm tools such as secular law, political support, and other similar secular weapons. People also pray.

Some problems are the lack of training in spiritual warfare and the poor familiarity with the Scriptures. The Scriptures form a foundation for each of the six spiritual weapons mentioned in Ephesians 6:10-18. Without a strong knowledge of Scripture and true wisdom, understanding, and knowledge, a person will have limited success in prevailing in any spiritual-realm skirmishes. There are more emphases and resources placed into the secular side of the effort than into training as in a spiritual boot camp. People have to become spiritual powers in order to influence these battle outcomes. To be powers, they have to develop their inner man under the tutorship of God. This is vastly different to developing intellectual and philosophical debating points. Only the degree of spiritual power a group can muster will determine who wins. Fortunately, the Lord multiples our efforts geometrically; and two can put to flight quite a large number (Leviticus 26:8).

In order to win the spiritual skirmishes, the Church must focus on the weapons God has given it and develop them in all of the body; and it must perform the battle in the spiritual realm.

In order to win, we have to know the character of God, His power, and the power of His angels. This combination far exceeds the power of the demonic forces. If the people of God could see this reality in the spiritual realm, they would concentrate on using spiritual weapons (2 Kings 6:17). The devil can defeat men when they operate against him in the secular realm; he is the prince of it. God may not be willing to help us as much in the natural realm; although He sometimes does it out of mercy. Clearly He wants us to join with Him in the spiritual realm. Our enemies are not men, whom evil spirits outmaneuver. Our enemies are in high places, and it is from there that we have to rout them; but it must always be as we follow the Lord God and know exactly His wishes for us in every individual skirmish. We should not initiate skirmishes; that is up to God.

14. Eternity

God tells us that He designed man to live with future eternal expectations.

Ecclesiastes 3:11

[11] He hath made every *thing* beautiful in his time: also he hath set the world in their heart, so that no man can find out the work that God maketh from the beginning to the end.

The Hebrew for *world* in this Scripture is much more often translated as ever, everlasting, perpetual, and evermore.

The Church is good about promoting the concept of eternal life with God after one obtains his gift of salvation. However, there is much left out about the experience for those who have been through the second birth and who have not been obedient to God. Many people do not seek God's purposes for themselves in all situations in their lives. Most people expecting to spend eternity in God's Kingdom assume that after death they will be face to face with the Lord. This is so, but there are many other considerations about which people should be taught. The following Scriptures make this clear.

2 Timothy 2:20

[20] But in a great house there are not only vessels of gold and of silver, but also of wood and of earth; and some to honour, and some to dishonour.

1 Corinthians 3:13–15

[13] Every man's work shall be made manifest: for the day shall declare it, because it shall be revealed by fire; and the fire shall try every man's work of what sort it is. [14] If any man's work abide which he hath built thereupon, he shall receive a reward. [15] If any man's work shall be burned, he shall suffer loss: but he himself shall be saved; yet so as by fire.

Eternity is a very long time and people deserve to know their options in order to make choices. It may not be a topic that some people will be pleased to hear BUT God says that:

2 Timothy 3:16

[16] All scripture *is* given by inspiration of God, and *is* profitable for doctrine, for reproof, for correction, for instruction in righteousness:

The Church needs to train people in the local churches in all of the Scriptures. People need to understand that their behavior in this phase of life limits options for them in eternity.

15. Educational goals and issues in the Church

One major cause of secularization in the Church comes through the unthinking adoption into the Church of the educational ideas in the natural realm in which teachers and administrators (many of whom may not have been through the second birth) set the curriculum and the depth of discussions. In this realm only highlights of various subjects are taught and the teacher assumes responsibility for the content of the education.

The Spiritual realm approach should be that all Scripture should be taught to all people. It is not just the ability of the teacher, but equally or more important is the heart of the hearer as to what is heard and the consequences of this. The teacher should be the vehicle of the Holy Spirit who will guide the topics and discussion when one is submitted to Him. It is God who should set the syllabus at each local church. A teacher should be able not only to teach principles but also to help individuals to operationalize God's Word into their lives. All too often we hear people teaching and preaching about what people should be like at the end of a process; but few teach how to bring about the required changes through operationalizing the Scriptures according to the plans that God has placed in His Word.

One common educational issue in the Church is the lack of adequately prepared teachers who understand spiritual-realm structure and function. Few teachers have their knowledge of Scripture founded on true wisdom, understanding, and knowledge. Even so, when God's Word goes forth, it will accomplish His purposes (Isaiah 55:11).

Churches need educational programs that cover the entire Word of God and that mentor people in relating to God and to His Word. Discipleship is very important for mentoring.

16. Secularization of the knowledge of the structure of man leaves out the impact of sin on health.

The Scriptures explain how God made man (body + spirit = soul [the individual]). It is very important that the structure of man be taught to Church members because it highlights the dual spiritual and natural components of man. By promoting it, we bring a greater awareness of truth.

The promotion of truth in any area of the creation is important. This is even more so in understanding the structure of man and how man functions. The Church needs to emphasize the impact of sin on our physical well being within both the Church and the community. The understanding of the relationship between sin and health does carry significant information for all people. The following two Scriptures are worth reviewing; they are complementary to each other.

Matthew 9:2–6

[2] And, behold, they brought to him a man sick of the palsy, lying on a bed: and Jesus seeing their faith said unto the sick of the palsy; Son, be of good cheer; thy sins be forgiven thee. [3] And, behold, certain of the scribes said within themselves, This *man* blasphemeth. [4] And Jesus knowing their thoughts said, Wherefore think ye evil in your hearts? [5] For whether is easier, to say, *Thy* sins be forgiven thee; or to say, Arise, and walk? [6] But that ye may know that the Son of man hath power on earth to forgive sins, (then saith he to the sick of the palsy,) Arise, take up thy bed, and go unto thine house.

John 9:1–3

[1] And as *Jesus* passed by, he saw a man which was blind from *his* birth. [2] And his disciples asked him, saying, Master, who did sin, this man, or his parents, that he was born blind? [3] Jesus answered, Neither hath this man sinned, nor his parents: but that the works of God should be made manifest in him.

In the Matthew passage there is a very direct link between illness and healing and with sins and forgiveness. In the John passage there is no similar link. There are a number of good reasons why this blindness was present from a natural-realm perspective; one is that this physical impairment might have been from a birth injury; it could have been genetically related; a familial spirit could have caused the blindness (which would be seen only with a spiritual-realm perspective). Regardless of the cause in this person, it is a fact that all illness has come about from the sin of Adam and Eve. The carrying of the sin nature has been genetically transmitted by the male since then.

These Scriptures show the complexity of understanding healing and illness in the Scriptures and why it is so hard to make any general rules. One can conclude that many times sin and illness are highly correlated; and even natural-realm observations bear this out in terms of the correlation of illness with behaviors that are called sinful in Scripture. One can never predict, however, what God will do for any particular individual who approaches Him for healing. We have given approaches to seeking healing from God which will make it likely to occur for a person who has been through the second birth. There are two groups of those who have not been through a second birth. The first is composed of those who have not been through a second birth but who think they have. The second is composed of those who do not think they have been through the second birth. In both cases one must believe in God to have a chance that he will be healed of a particular problem. The Scripture below addresses these issues.

Hebrews 11:6

⁶ But without faith *it is* impossible to please *him*: for he that cometh to God must believe that he is, and *that* he is a rewarder of them that diligently seek him.

In addition, there are circumstances in which one's prayers might be hindreed. If one is aware of any sin, he would be well advised to confess it and seek forgiveness in order that his prayers not be hindered. The Scriptures below discuss several situations in which God will not listen to one's requests.

1 Peter 3:7

[7] Likewise, ye husbands, dwell with *them* according to knowledge, giving honour unto the wife, as unto the weaker vessel, and as being heirs together of the grace of life; that your prayers be not hindered.

Matthew 5:24

[24] Leave there thy gift before the altar, and go thy way; first be reconciled to thy brother, and then come and offer thy gift.

Isaiah 59:1–2

[1] Behold, the LORD'S hand is not shortened, that it cannot save; neither his ear heavy, that it cannot hear: [2] But your iniquities have separated between you and your God, and your sins have hid *his* face from you, that he will not hear.

The present Church in the West has some similarity to the Church in Laodicea (Revelation 3:14-22)

Secularization and the Church of Laodicea

The Church in the West has failed to provide the community with the knowledge of God's commands, His power, and His character. Many churches have been involved in healing using secular approaches to health care, including providing clinics and hospitals. There is nothing wrong with this; indeed, it is commendable. The problem is that these secularized Church-sponsored forays into providing health care in the community do not focus on the potential for a person to receive a better healing directly from God. If God's people showed this to the community, then it would be noticed; and it would also bring economic benefit. Since health care is a major concern for many people, then we lose a great opportunity to reveal God to the local community. There are other major areas of life (finances, relationships, and family) in which the church has endorsed secular thinking, resulting in lost opportunities to show God's power, His abilities, and His character to the community. God's solutions in all of these areas are much better than secular solutions. This secularization of the church in the community greatly weakens the present-day church in the West. It is diagnostic of a suboptimal relationship with the head of the Church. It is alarmingly consistent with the prevailing beliefs that were present in the Church of Laodicea; a concern is that God will do to the church in the West what He threatened to do to that in Laodicea.

Revelation 3:15–19

[15] I know thy works, that thou art neither cold nor hot: I would thou wert cold or hot. [16] So then because thou art lukewarm, and neither cold nor hot, I will spue thee out of my mouth. [17] Because thou sayest, I am rich, and increased with goods, and have need of nothing; and knowest not that thou art wretched, and miserable, and poor, and blind, and naked: [18] I counsel thee to buy of me gold tried in the fire, that thou mayest be rich; and white raiment, that thou mayest be clothed, and *that* the shame of thy nakedness do not appear; and anoint thine eyes with eyesalve, that thou mayest see. [19] As many as I love, I rebuke and chasten: be zealous therefore, and repent.

The people in Laodicea were depending on secular approaches from natural-realm wealth for their needs. Similarly, the current Church in the West depends on wealth of natural knowledge and financial wealth for its needs. In this generation the state provides health care in many countries, and people do not look to God for their needs. People tend to be very neutral in their seeking of God; they are neither hot nor cold.

While there are some similarities to the Church in Laodicea, there are also differences.

While the Church in the West appears somewhat similar to that of the Church at Laodicea, there are differences in the spiritual realm. The present church is obviously larger and more heterogenous in many aspects than a relatively small local city church. Within the Church in the West there are many "tares," people that God does not know. Many of these people assume they have received salvation when they have not. There are also many true members who have been through the second birth.

Some of those people who have been through the second birth and who are in leadership positions have been through trying times. Many have wounded spirits and heavy hearts, weighed down by constant demonic assaults on their church members, their families, and themselves. The demons have been used to winning battles the last four hundred years. They have grown impudent; they are in one's face; and they are bold and brazen.

The last four hundred years have not been very good for the church. While there have been victories for the church in the constant spiritual war, they have been few and far between. There are some signs that this is about to change. God wants people in His Church who will commit to maturing in their relationship with Him. God wants the Church to be victorious. There are many who are in leadership and who need spiritual healing; after healing God will be able to use them mightily.

God wants to unleash His enormously powerful Spirit of Love on these people, carried by anointed servants, in order to heal them. All steps toward spiritual maturation in local churches need to be done in the Spirit of Love. God will then be able to give the Church a pathway to victory for a season before the final falling of the church into apostasy at the end of the age.

Jeremiah 9:24 - 10:17

Recently, the Lord has seemed to indicate that the issues Jeremiah was discussing in these Scriptures are pertinent for the near future. If so, this will be exciting and challenging for the Church; it will be a time of great opportunity. We will wait for more clarification from God.

In reading these Scriptures we see that God is calling His people to be separated and holy. We are to be separated from current idols such as the worship of false wisdom, understanding, and knowledge. We are to be separated from lures of the material.

Jeremiah 10:17

17 Gather up thy wares out of the land, O inhabitant of the fortress.

If God's people will not heed His call to be holy, then they will be punished, just as Israel was to be punished (Jeremiah 9:24-10:17).

Jeremiah 9:25

25 Behold, the days come, saith the LORD, that I will punish all them which are circumcised with the uncircumcised;

God's purposes for the creation

We have looked at God's purposes for creation in earlier chapters. Many of the parables are based on farming analogies—to have a good crop grow and to reap a good harvest (Matthew 13:39 [below], Mark 4:29, and Luke 10:2). There is also a theme running through Scripture comparing birth pains with the beginnings of a new phase of God's plans. Isaiah 66:9, Ezekiel 16:3, Galatians 4:19, and Revelation 12:2 illustrate this.

Matthew 13:39

39 The enemy that sowed them is the devil; the harvest is the end of the world; and the reapers are the angels.

Since many Scriptures do portray birth pains, Bruce was not surprised when he was shown the present age as a womb that is greatly diseased. The Church must work with God to bring many to birth through these very adverse circumstances in which gestation will occur. To do this, the Church must carry the Spirit of God in all the power of this Spirit into the environment. After the second birth culminating from these gestations, the Church should nurture each new creation in the presence of the Lord God, using His power. The goal is for the new children of God to grow to the point where they too can carry the Spirit of God in full power, and so to be salt and light in their surroundings.

The question then becomes how one gets from the present state of a dysfunctional church to that of a Church filled with God's power, love, joy, and peace which it can broadcast into communities around the world. The answer is in the Scriptures. We will review the aspects of it below.

God's solutions for healing the Church in the West

We are including this section here for completeness. It will be brief, and we will not elaborate much on the principles. The first model we will look at is the Church of Laodicea.

God provides these solutions for the current secularization of the Church in the West in the Scripture printed above about the Church in Laodicea. They are totally opposite from the secular way the Church in the West functions. We will compare these points below (taken from the Scripture about the Church in Laodicea) with the equivalent points revealed by the Lord God in points 1 to 16 earlier in this chapter.

1. Find leaders who have been through the fire instead of those with just secular qualifications—which the Church in the West currently seeks. The fire is through significant trials God has allowed to develop an individual.

2. Seek spiritual riches (not natural-realm riches—this involves seeking God and the relationship with Him).

3. Become purified in heart and Holy in order to wear white (Revelation 3:18). We have discussed how to become purified in the heart earlier. Holiness involves separation from any desires for natural-realm goods and gains. God may give some of these, but we should not desire them.

4. Have spiritual salve placed on your eyes to open your spiritual sense of vision—focus on the spiritual realm for inspiration in which to work in the natural realm.

5. Become zealous for righteousness and obedience to God by getting to know Him and to love Him above all else

6. Repent; and in repenting, restore the time and resources robbed from God through earlier behavior

Some further Scriptures are pertinent to the above discussion:

1 Corinthians 2:14–15

[14] But the natural man receiveth not the things of the Spirit of God: for they are foolishness unto him: neither can he know *them*, because they are spiritually discerned. [15] But he that is spiritual judgeth all things, yet he himself is judged of no man.

The net result of operating in the natural realm is a poor knowledge of God. It is very important to note that the poor knowledge of God is not the same as not learning a lot about God. The Pharisees studied the Scriptures frequently and intensively, and yet they missed major truths including who the Lord Jesus Christ is. Pharisaical types of false doctrine are prevalent in the church because they are derived from secular reasoning.

The following Scriptures show this.

John 5:39–40

[39] Search the scriptures; for in them ye think ye have eternal life: and they are they which testify of me. [40] And ye will not come to me, that ye might have life.

The Sadducees also had the same problem.

Mark 12:24–27

[24] And Jesus answering said unto them, Do ye not therefore err, because ye know not the scriptures, neither the power of God? [25] For when they shall rise from the dead, they neither marry, nor are given in marriage; but are as the angels which are in heaven. [26] And as touching the dead, that they rise: have ye not read in the book of Moses, how in the bush God spake unto him, saying, I *am* the God of Abraham, and the God of Isaac, and the God of Jacob? [27] He is not the **God** of the dead, but the God of the living: ye therefore do greatly err.

The problem with false doctrine in the Church

There is much false doctrine taught, mainly unthinkingly, in churches today because people (including pastors) generally do not study the Scriptures carefully and completely under the influence of the Holy Spirit. This problem is more prevalent in some denominations than in others. It is only as one reads Scripture and lets the Holy Spirit point out deeper things every time he reads through them that such false doctrine can be eliminated. .

God wants all of His people, not just an occasional person here and there, continually studying His entire Word (not just a cursory reading of the Word) in order to be equipped. Taking God's Word as a medicine several times daily heals diseases and strengthens the spirit greatly (Proverbs 4:22).

Our Great God

Psalm 147:5

[5] Great *is* our Lord, and of great power: his understanding *is* in-

finite.

This really says it all. His power is impossible to imagine, His attention span, His memory, His ability to see to the very bottom of every human heart, His ability to judge justly, His future plans and prophecies, and many other things point to His unsearchable greatness. Unfortunately, very little understanding of this seems to be present in the hearts of the people of the Church. They know of God and some things about God, but they scarcely know God.

After going to many churches over many years, we have neither heard nor read in publications and books any systematic attempt to help people come to know this great God who shares His emotions freely and who shares practical advice with His people who ask. One minor example of getting practical advice that well illustrates this was a time the authors had a problem deciding how to handle an office dispute between two employees. After prayer the feeling of God's peace flooded Bruce's heart. Bruce implemented the advice promptly, and the situation was resolved amicably. If only we would all call on the Lord with all of our problems, our local churches would be filled with people seeking God's help.

We are not being critical of any person or group. We are trying to sound an alarm, for we feel that God's Church in the West is failing to be what He wishes it to be. He is kind and patient, but He expects more than He is getting. No individual or single group of people is responsible for the present situation, which has evolved over four hundred years of gradual slipping under the subterfuges of the evil spirits. The overall spiritual paucity has come about by the very deceptive wiles and machines of the devil and his philosophies, which have gradually been taken into the church. God will not use these. They result in the fruit of death, regardless of how good they look. God and the world need a spiritually mature Church. God is the healer, and He will heal His Church; He will not choose another plan. Those who obstruct His plans will have difficulties in the coming changes

Final Statements

Some practical issues when seeking healing from God

This book is about spiritual and physical healing that God can and will provide under circumstances which meet His approval. All transactions for divine healing have to be one on one with God. There is almost always a spiritual illness that will need to be corrected in order for God to bless with healing.

None of us knows the depth of the content of our own heart; and we certainly cannot speak about another person's heart. Some sin patterns are obvious, and one can advise in that case; but in the issues of not listening to God, not being obedient to Him in all of the small communication issues, and similar hard to detect attitudes, one may not able to advise another person.

The devil can perceive so readily what a person's motivation for seeking healing is. If a person has spiritual pride, it is less likely that God will bless him with healing. Evil spirits can also deceive a person about his state of health. Some people have religious spirits which try to block them from seeking healing.

When one is seeking healing from God, it is wise to have a physician monitor the situation.

The Spiritual Poverty of the Church

The people of God can and must address the spiritual poverty of the Church. It is going to take spiritually mature leaders, not just people with spiritual gifting, to work closely with God under His leadership to bring the Church in the West back to being salt and light in the communities in which it is found.

We live in a spiritually poor time, and there are some very specific strategies one can bring into operation to improve this. God will continue to reveal His plans for restoring the Church, for this is His intent.

Steps we need to take as individuals and corporately:

1.   Acknowledge the truth of the spiritual paucity (a critical first step) and repent (making an immediate change in direction and redeeming the time, and lost resources).

2.   Promote widely the need for renewing the mind, taking thoughts captive and purifying the hearts of all individuals.

3.   Promote widely the consequences eternally of not being pleasing to God (loss of reward and eternal condemnation).

4.   Teach and mentor how to learn to communicate with God and how not to be deceived by evil spirits.

5.   Get the concept of eternity into the hearts of the people.

6.   Mentor people in how to grow in spiritual strength and wisdom.

7.   Change the structure of individual churches to include more focus on the spiritual teaching methods—revelation, prophecy, word of knowledge, true doctrine, and power.

8.   Reveal the magnitude and greatness of God's character and His power.

9.   Teach widely the plans God has for His creation.

10.   Join God in determining plans to take back the works of the spirit of knowledge, which has gone largely unchecked for four hundred years. This is going to require a completely spiritual-realm focus in order to succeed in the natural realm.

This is not a complete list but is included rather as a guide to future plans. There is no time to waste, however. God can direct a strategy for each of the above items.

What complete healing will look like

God is looking for restoration of the intimate friendship that He had with Adam and Eve prior to their fall. Sin always makes a person hide from God, as witnessed by the reaction of Adam and Eve (Genesis 3:8-10).

When a person has left all of his sin patterns behind he will seek intimacy with God instead of seeking to perform work for God. He will want to be with God and spend time enjoying the presence of the love, the peace, the joy, and the power which fill him. His first desire will be to have this rich and close fellowship. Out of this relationship God will provide work for him.

Many times God allows work for Him by an individual to bring about the more mature relationship. When we have no sin, we have confidence toward God, as described in 1 John 3:21 and 1 John 5:14.

When we have this deep confidence in God, we know that He will hear us and that He will heal us of our diseases for His glory. It may take time for the healing to be complete.

May God richly bless all of the people who read this book.

To God be the Glory; great things hath he done, and what great things He will do!

Jude 24–25

[24] Now unto him that is able to keep you from falling, and to present you faultless before the presence of his glory with exceeding joy, [25] To the only wise God our Saviour, be glory and majesty, dominion and power, both now and ever. Amen.

www.ingramcontent.com/pod-product-compliance
Lightning Source LLC
Chambersburg PA
CBHW071538200326
41519CB00021BB/6529